the healing
POWER OF EXERCISE

AN ANTHOLOGY BY
PAT ROBINSON

Front cover design by
Emma Kelly Photography, http://www.emmakelly.co.uk

Photographs of Ben Saunders by
Richard Blake (top) and Martin Hartley (bottom) page 16

Published by:
Best Global Publishing Ltd
PO Box 9633
Brentwood
Essex
CM13 1ZT
United Kingdom

Dedication

For my parents and my son Tom.

Contents

Introduction

THE HEALING POWER OF EXERCISE

I compiled this anthology in the hope that it would inspire others and to show that even if you have reached rock bottom mentally, as some of the contributors to this book have, there is a way upwards without having to permanently resort to artificial mood enhancing stimulants that only give short-term comfort and temporary oblivion.

Obviously there are cases where it is necessary for doctors to prescribe anti-depressants, but relying just on drugs long term is not the only answer. I know because I've been there and know that exercise can help you overcome depression and it can be a long-term solution.

Numerous books have been written about depression in particular, but I wanted to obtain anecdotal evidence of the enormous benefits that exercise can give you, both mentally and physically. These stories are from ordinary people, of all ages, all sizes and all races and they all confirm that taking up exercise can be life enhancing.

Some of the people who have contributed to this anthology talk about being stressed, having little or no confidence, poor self-image, dependency on drugs and/or alcohol and, because of these negative feelings, this has culminated in bouts of depression.

Depression is one of the most common health problems of modern times. At least one in six of us are likely to suffer from it at some point in our lives. For some the effects are crippling; low mood, anxiety, tearfulness, short temper, insomnia, exhaustion, lack of appetite, reduced libido, withdrawing and cutting off from social situations, all of which make it hard to function well in day to day life. Increasingly, doctors have been relying on drugs to fix the problem. Prescriptions for anti-depressants have almost tripled in the past ten years.

A growing body of research suggests that exercise may be a better prescription for people with mild to moderate depression. So persuasive is this evidence that the National Institute for Clinical Excellence, which provides professionals with guidelines on patient care, advises GPs to inform mildly depressed patients about exercise as a form of treatment. This fact is born out by some of the contributors to this book who were referred to the YMCA gym by their doctor.

Research shows that exercising three to five times a week for at least half an hour releases feel-good hormones called endorphins, producing a natural euphoria. Experts also believe that exercise stimulates brain cell regeneration and gives patients a sense of purpose. It also provides a chance to meet people, further helping to overcome depression.

A study in the United States looked at three groups of patients with mild to moderate depression. One group took anti-depressants, the second used only exercise as a treatment and the third used a combination of drugs and exercise. Positive effects were greatest in the group that used only exercise in their treatment.

Whilst any type of exercise – from weight training to walking – seems to have a beneficial affect, experts recommend regular aerobic exercise at about 70% of your maximum capacity, for at least twenty to thirty minutes per session, for the best mood-lifting benefits. Obviously the physical benefits are manifold; regular exercise will strengthen your immune system, give you a healthier body, a stronger heart, a hardier skeleton, a lower risk of cancer, a better body image and a longer life. Looking and feeling better will inevitably make you feel more confident.

The healing power of exercise, therefore, is obvious and doctors are now referring more patients with anxiety and depression to the gym.

Many contributors say that they found it difficult to get started. Unfortunately, with the pace of modern life, many people want a quick fix. Nothing of real long-term benefit will come easy, like the push of a button on a remote control. If you have to put effort into achieving a goal then the rewards are well worth the struggle, as is confirmed by the contributors to this anthology. This book is about ordinary people who have enhanced their lives through regular exercise. All you need is a pair of trainers and the determination to get started.

Pat Robinson

Acknowledgements

Jamie Beverton, for his unfailing friendship and support.

Emma Kelly, Emma Kelly Photography, for book cover design and cover photographs of Pat Robinson.

Dr Kaur, for her constant support.

YMCA Health and Fitness Club, Nottingham.

Holme Pierrepont Running Club.

Mike Mills, Jacobs, Nottingham.

Tom Anson, CD Republic, Nottingham.

And to all the people in this book who have shared their stories.

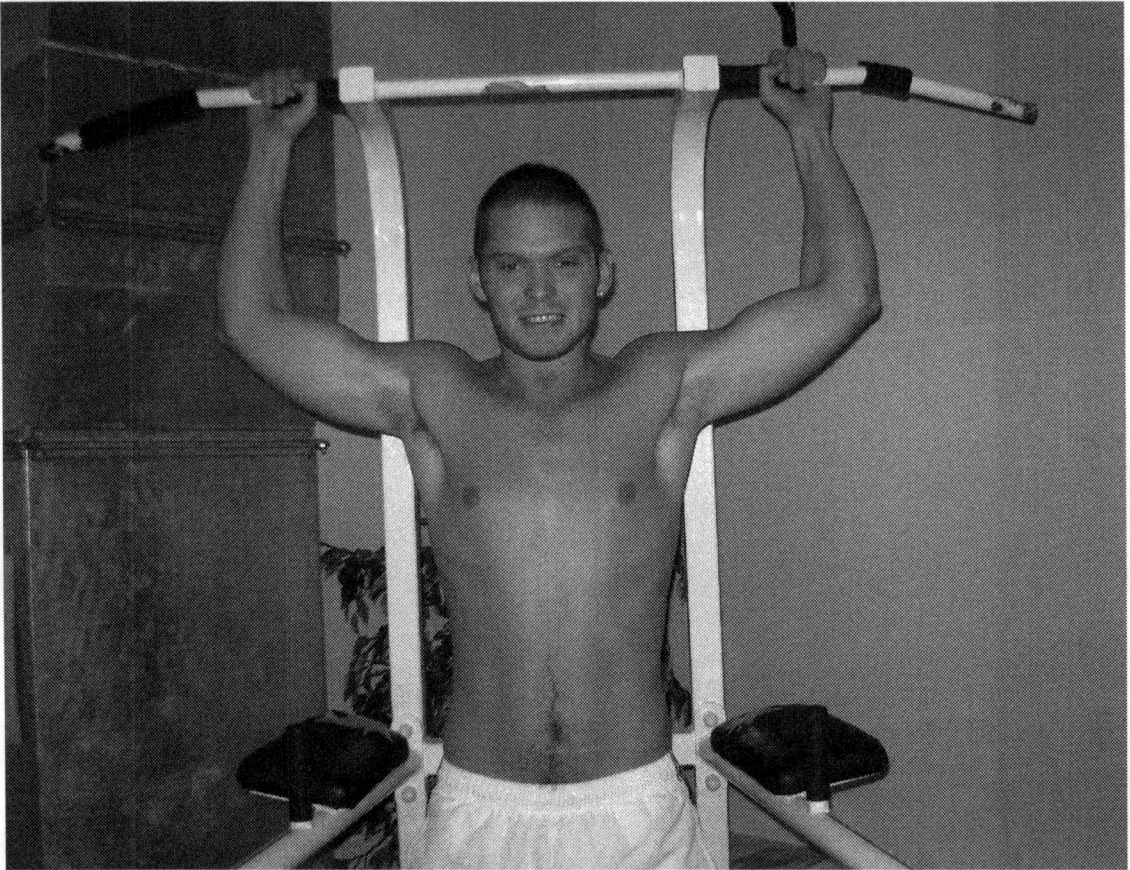

Adam Tells His Story

I was pretty skinny when I was younger. I used to play football but pulled a ligament so I couldn't play anymore. My mate's dad suggested I join a gym, which I did. I started weight training and enjoyed pushing myself and started to notice that my body was getting toned.

I was depressed in the job I was in. It wasn't fulfilling. I wanted to train and get involved in a job in the fitness industry. I now have a job at the YMCA gym and enjoy my work as a personal trainer. I've seen real changes in people who come in to train regularly.

Whenever I get down, I train in the gym and it lifts me. I still like to push myself and set new challenges. Achieving new challenges makes me feel good, physically and mentally.

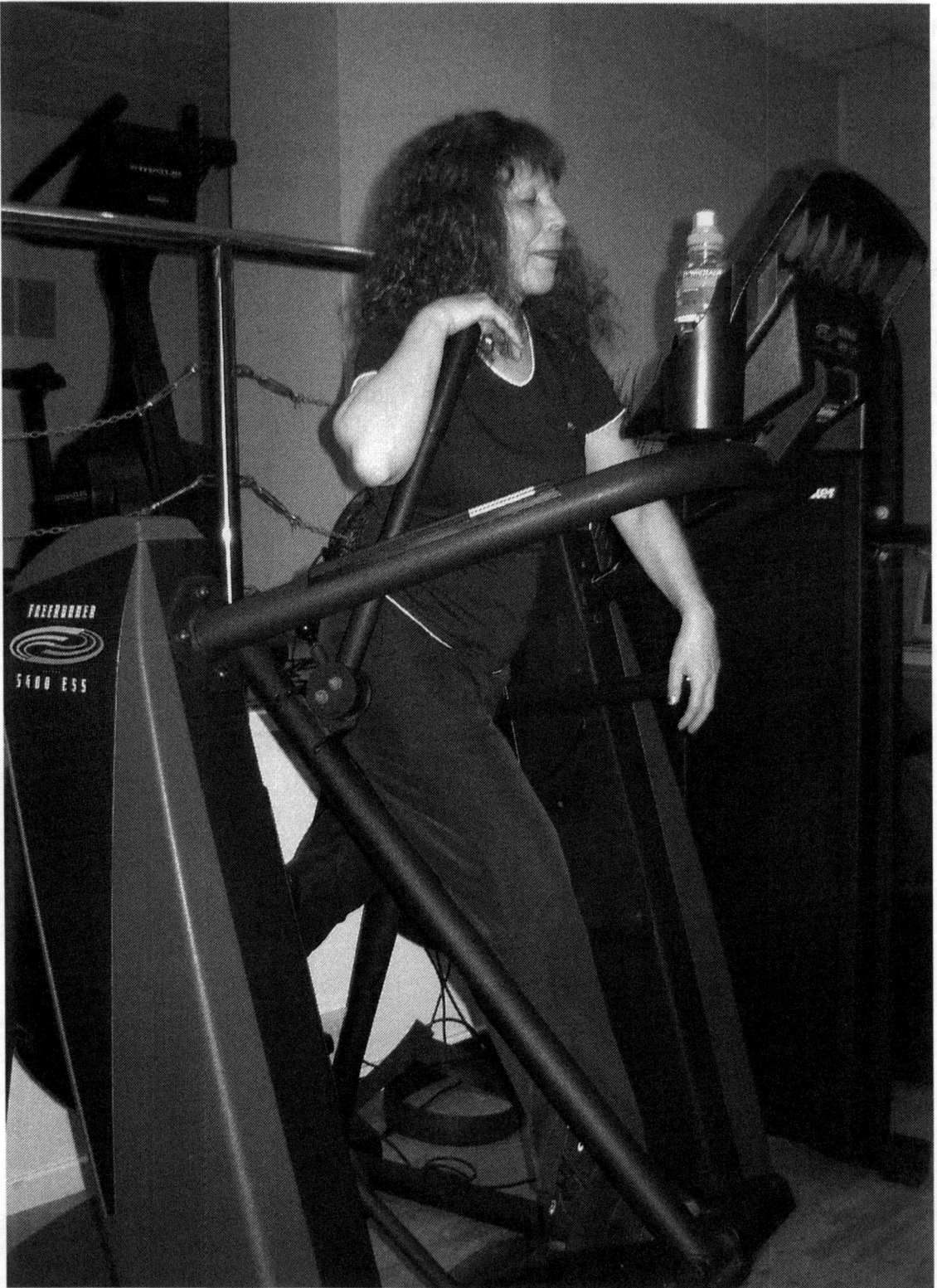

Anne-Kine Tells Her Story

I've been exercising on a regular basis for more than thirty years. Exercising makes me feel great, both physically and mentally. I get a lot of energy from it and it's a great stress release after my working day! Being fit also keeps me healthy and strong. I also think it's fun to exercise to music!

Miscellaneous Stories from YMCA Gym Members

"I hated sports when I was a kid. My aversion to school sports was so strong that I'd do anything to avoid it, from forging sick notes to feigning illness on the pitch. The problem was that I was always very restless, and instead of channelling my energy into healthy pursuits like sports, I started drinking alcohol and dabbling with various drugs. This started at about the age of twelve and really started becoming a serious problem after leaving school at sixteen. I drifted from one dead end job to another, with long periods of unemployment in between. I only associated with people who abused alcohol. I was often depressed and was always on some sort of psychiatric medication for depression.

After several unsuccessful attempts to stop drinking, and several hospital admissions, which included treatment, I finally managed to stop altogether when I was thirty-two. I suddenly had loads of spare time and so I joined the YMCA gym in Nottingham. I started attending regularly and found that I really enjoyed it. After a year of attending the gym a fellow member suggested that I try running and introduced me to a club. On the first day I went for a six mile run around Holme Pierrpont in Nottingham and I experienced the 'runner's high' for the first time. It was a wonderful experience and I have not looked back ever since.

Competitive running has completely changed my attitude towards competitive sports and teamwork. Besides getting me really physically fit, it has also strengthened my character, given me a more positive and resilient attitude, and it has helped me remain totally free from alcohol and drugs. I have learned the hard way that real, genuine pleasure comes from overcoming life's numerous hurdles and difficulties. Vigorous exercise can be hard to begin with but the rewards are immense and so the effort is well worth it."

"I never liked doing exercise. I found it too hard. I always hated doing it at school, which you just had to do! As an adult, my doctor referred me to the YMCA gym because I was depressed. I was put on a programme by the personal trainers. I found it hard at first, but I persevered. I'd nothing to lose. I'd tried everything else. Anyway, it got easier. Now exercise is part of my life. It's so true that a fitter body will make you feel more confident and this will make you have a 'fitter' mind. I would definitely say that exercise has changed my life, for the better."

"I always had a burning rage. I hated myself. I started doing martial arts and found that I was able to channel this rage. I began training seriously eight years ago and I have never looked back."

"I've always exercised. Exercise is the way I deal with stress. When I've done a good workout, I feel good."

"I've always had an eating problem. Nobody understands that it is a problem. People look down upon you when you are overweight. I was very overweight – obese – but I could not stop overeating. It was a way that I dealt with depression. It was comfort eating. But, obviously, it was a vicious circle because in the end you become more depressed when you see yourself getting bigger. My health was suffering too.

Anyway, I joined the YMCA gym and they put me on a programme. I still struggle with my overeating for comfort, but since being put on the programme I have lost weight and now try to do regular exercise. I have also bought a pedometer and make sure that I do plenty of walking each day."

"Training is really important to me. I'd feel sluggish without it. Exercise always makes me feel positive."

"I was never happy with my image, but since I have started doing regular exercise, I feel so much more confident."

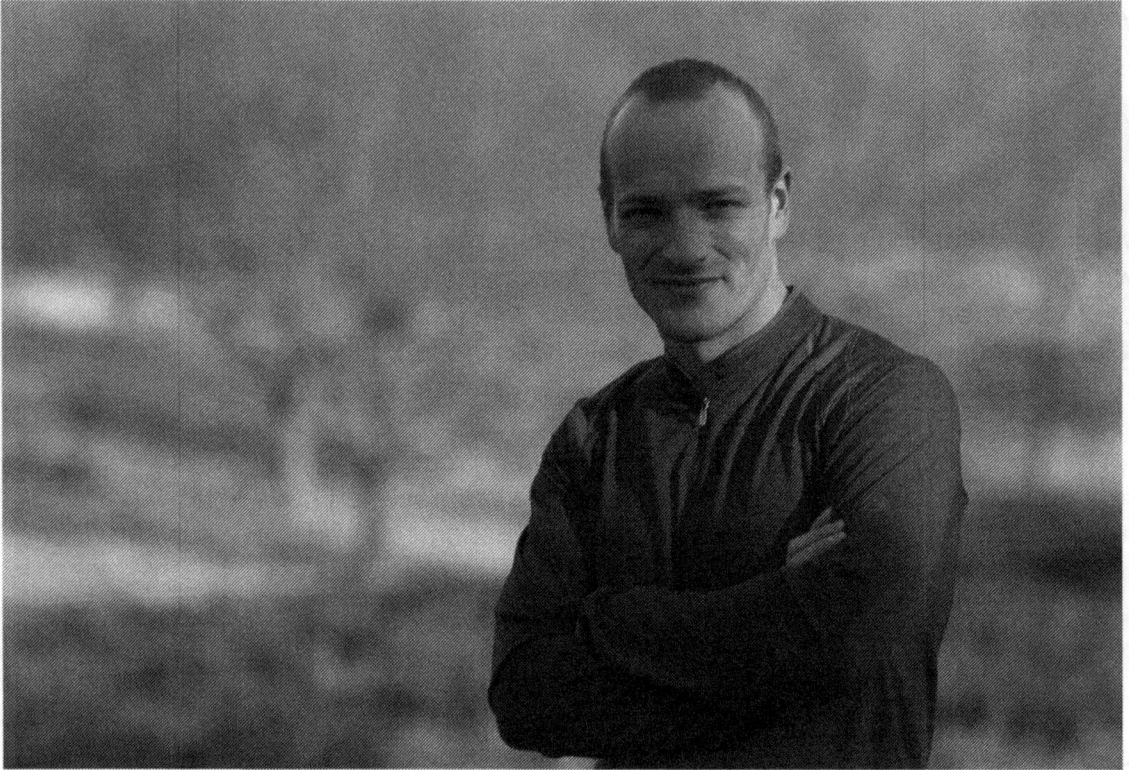

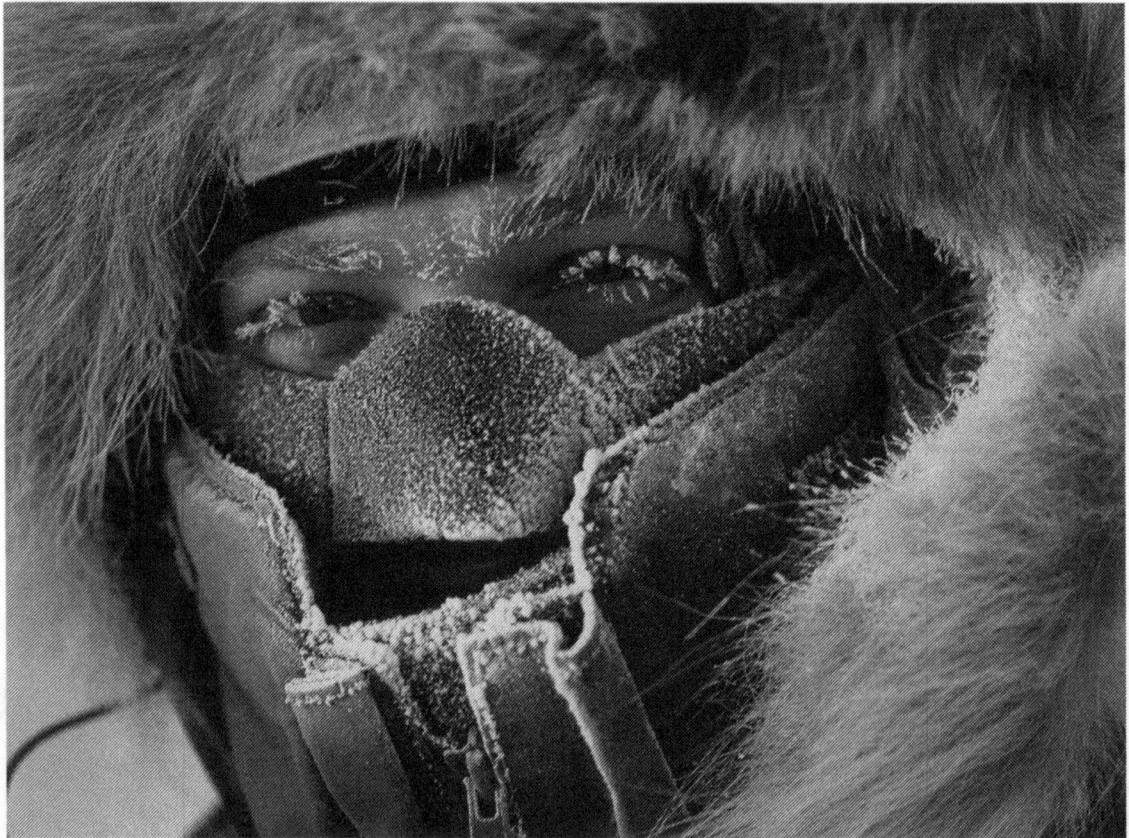

Ben Tells His Story

I was the podgy kid at school that was always picked last for the football team. When I was thirteen one teacher wrote on my school report, 'Ben lacks sufficient impetus to achieve anything worthwhile.' I firmly believe that everyone is capable of achieving his or her ambitions, no matter how steep the odds. Much depends on goal setting and teamwork. Success, failure, risk-taking and overcoming adversity are all part of the challenge. I am so passionate in this belief that I spend much of my time - when not skiing or pulling a sledge across the Arctic - working as a motivational speaker, with audiences ranging from primary school children to board-level directors of some of the world's largest multinationals.

After an unpromising start at school, I discovered mountain biking in my teens and went on to race bikes on and off-road at national level. I have run several marathons (New York is my favourite course and 2 hours 55 minutes is my best time to date), two ultra marathons, and I aim to start competing in Ironman distance triathlons before too long.

Skiing and Arctic exploration are the real driving forces in my life. When I was 19 I began working as an instructor at the John Ridgway School of Adventure in the Scottish Highlands. John became a role model and mentor of the highest calibre. In 1966 he and Chay Blyth rowed the Atlantic in an open boat, and John went on to break records in non-stop round the world sailing. It was then that I started planning my first expedition, inspired by the tremendous voyages of Ranulph Fiennes and Robert Swan.

In the past five years I have skied more than 2,500km. In 2004 I became the youngest person to ski solo to the North Pole and in doing so I broke the record for the longest solo Arctic journey by a Briton. It is, without doubt, one of the most challenging goals facing today's adventurers - the four-minute mile of the Arctic.

I am now preparing for SOUTH, a four-month trek that will be the first ever South Pole round trip on foot and the longest unsupported polar journey in history. Many experts still consider it to be impossible. Our team will have no outside assistance, no air resupplies and will ski every mile under our own motive power, man hauling 400lb sledges across 1,800 miles of the most hostile terrain on Earth, to the Pole and back. This expedition is about dreaming big. I would encourage everyone to have dreams, to take risks and to not fear failure.

Ben Saunders, record-breaking long-distance skier.

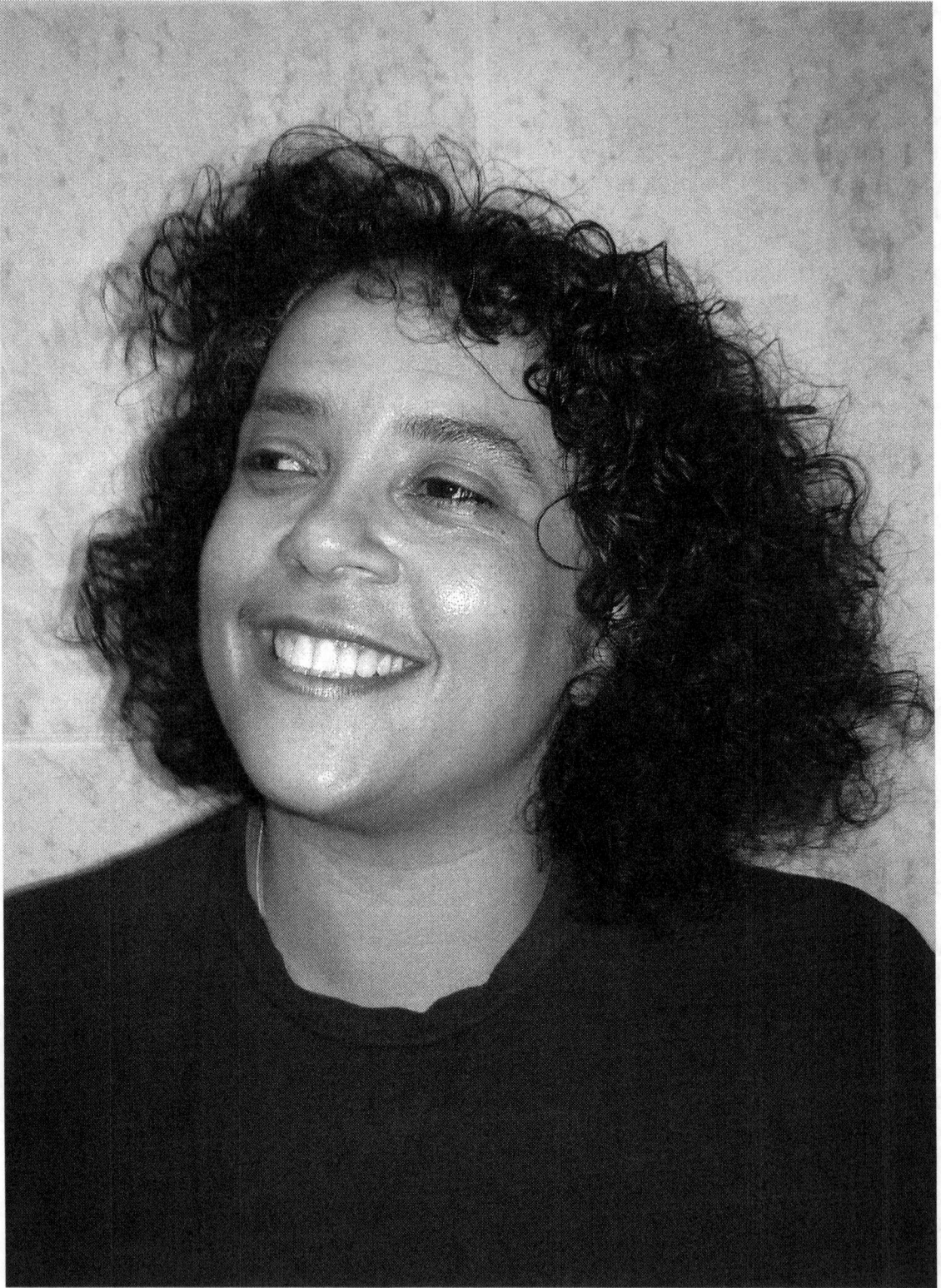

Carmen Tells Her Story

I took up exercise to deal with stress initially. I had suffered two bereavements and started comfort eating. My weight went up and my confidence went down. I had no confidence whatsoever and had a very poor self-image. I felt awful. Everything became a vicious circle. I was confident in my work and with friends, but not at all confident with my image.

I joined the YMCA gym and was given a programme to work on that involved using the treadmill and the exercise bike. I also started swimming. It was difficult at first, it still is, but it's getting easier. All I can say is that working out (exercise) takes away stress. I start to put things into perspective. When I exercise I always think of it as *my time*.

I have already lost four stone and hope to get down to the healthy weight I want to be soon. I feel much more confident now. I recommend regular exercise to everyone.

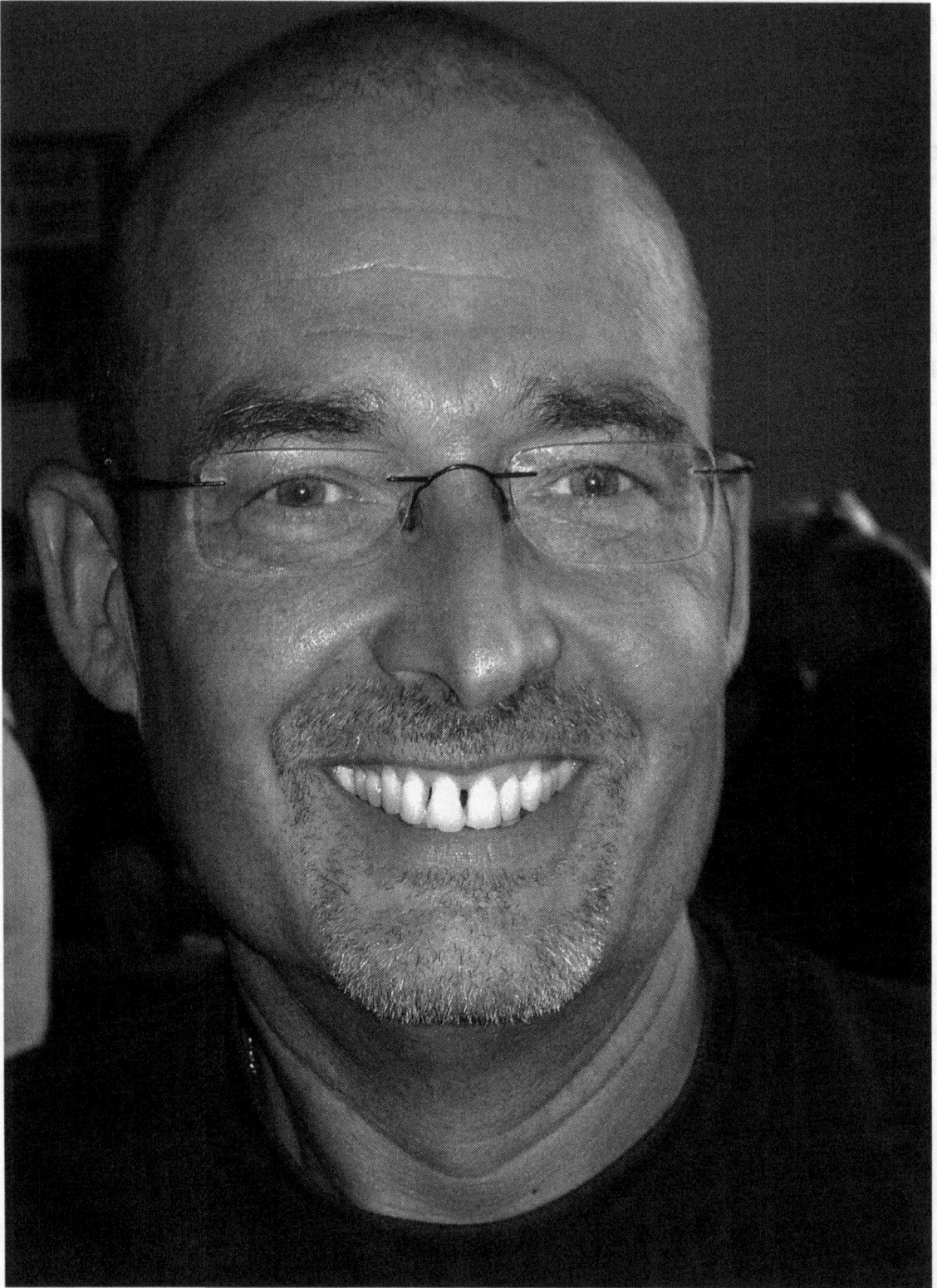

Chris Tells His Story

Nine years ago we were told that my grandson had leukaemia. It was a terrible shock. I decided to do something positive to deal with the helplessness that I felt when I heard the diagnosis. I decided to raise money for a leukaemia charity by running the London Marathon. I started training hard and this helped me deal with my grandson's illness. I felt great when I'd finished the marathon and nine years later I'm still running and racing.

The great news is that my grandson is now free of leukaemia, is strong and healthy and has also started running. We entered a race together recently and it was great to see him finish and get his medal.

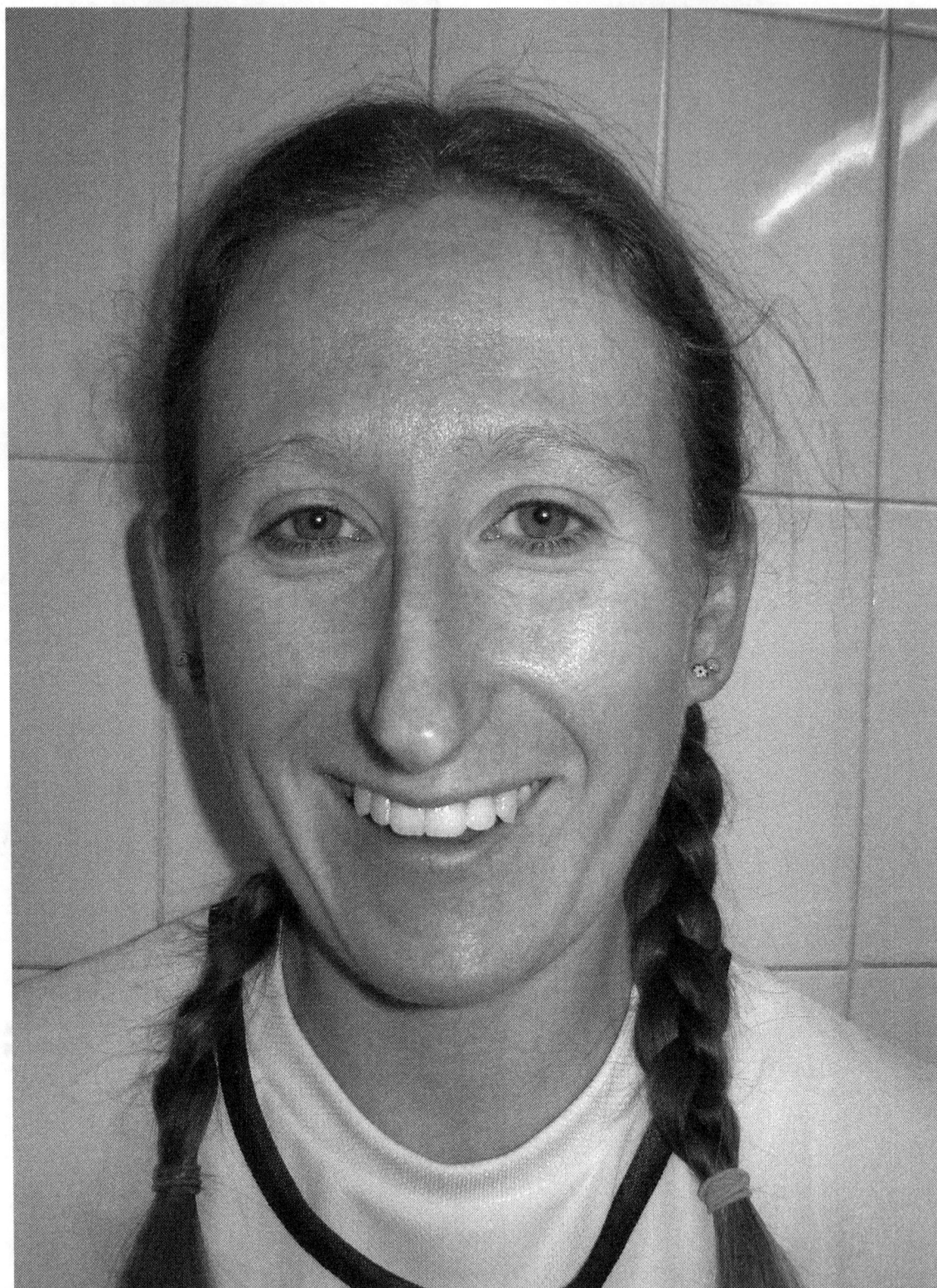

Claire Tells Her Story

Three years ago I never thought I would be able to run three miles, let alone the marathon that I have just completed.

When you run you can just forget about things that are stressing you. You can also think things through logically and just let all the stress fall away!

There is a great sense of achievement in keeping fit through running, both mental and physical. And I don't have to go to weight watchers; I can even eat chocolate now!

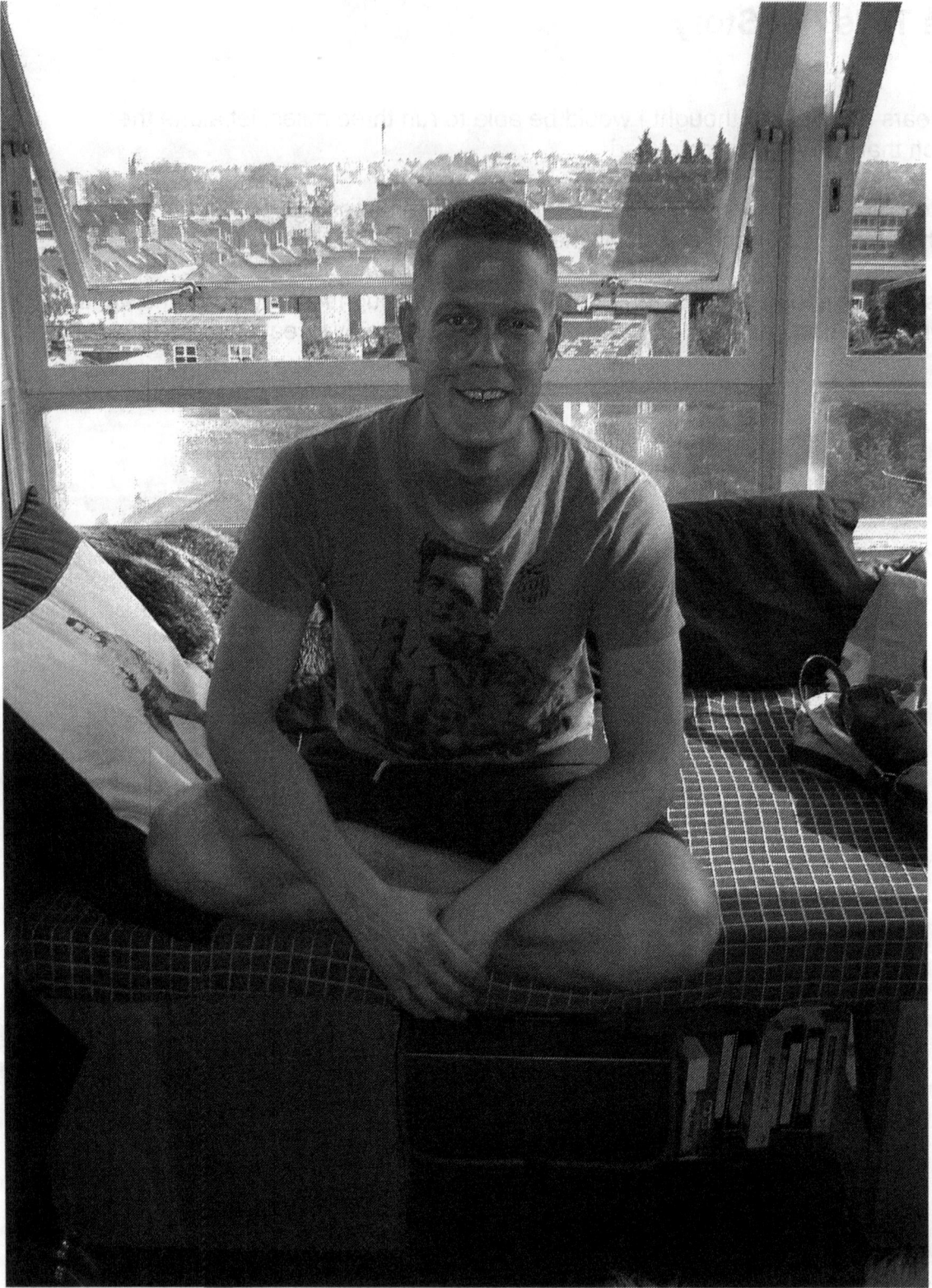

Clint Tells His Story

Just over six months ago I took part in a programme on BBC1 called *Run for Glory*. I was selected as one of thirteen people, all with a very different and often harrowing story, to train for just six months to run the London Marathon. This is my story before taking part in this challenge.

In 1997, when I was only 17, I found out that I was HIV positive. At first I thought I had cancer as the doctor had said I was low risk. I became very ill, losing two stone in weight, had night sweats, also general infections that affected my nerve endings. After months of not knowing what was wrong with me, I eventually had some tests done and was diagnosed as being HIV positive. In some strange way, although it was a terrible shock, it was a relief to eventually know what I was dealing with. Soon after testing positive, I rapidly developed AIDS and spent months in and out of hospital. I was very scared. I asked the doctor, "How long have I got to live?" He said I could have ten healthy years. I remember at the time thinking that that was better than having cancer as I had thought that my life expectancy would be shorter if I had.

'Positive Youth', the only HIV peer based charity in London, folded in 1997, the year I was diagnosed. To understand and learn more about HIV I became a volunteer for a charity called Oxaids. I realised that there were very few services in the UK in 1997 for young people to be tested and to meet others with HIV, except for an organisation called 'Body & Soul' which only dealt with young people up to 19 who were heterosexuals. There was no organisation that was inclusive of young homosexuals. After treatments, I went to America and worked voluntarily for a HIV charity. I also studied at the University of California and San Francisco. I wanted to challenge myself and eventually raise awareness about AIDS. I heard so many stories and thought, "I've been lucky. I have the support and love of my family, the opportunity to travel abroad and find out more about HIV." I wanted to share that with other young people who weren't so lucky in this country.

In the USA, services were targeted through young people's involvement and were accessible at weekends. I wanted the same services in the UK so, in 1999 I set up a charity called Health Initiatives (HI), to provide tailored services and training with accurate age appropriate information and counselling that motivates and empowers young people to take control of their lives when testing and living with HIV and AIDS. Our aim is to open the UK's only weekend HIV testing centre in London. So that is my story, prior to taking part in training for the London Marathon. It was so hard at first. I used to get out of breath just running a short distance, and then I started to enjoy running and feeling stronger and fitter. I enjoyed challenging myself. My life for the last nine years had just revolved around HIV and it was good to set myself a new, positive challenge.

I finished the marathon, even with an injury, in a reasonable time of 4 hours 26 minutes. My time was 1 hour 45 minutes half way but my leg injury stopped me from continuing at that pace. Taking up running has changed my life and my way of thinking. My immune system has improved and my body is coping very well. I have now joined a running club and can't wait to continue with my new found fitness.

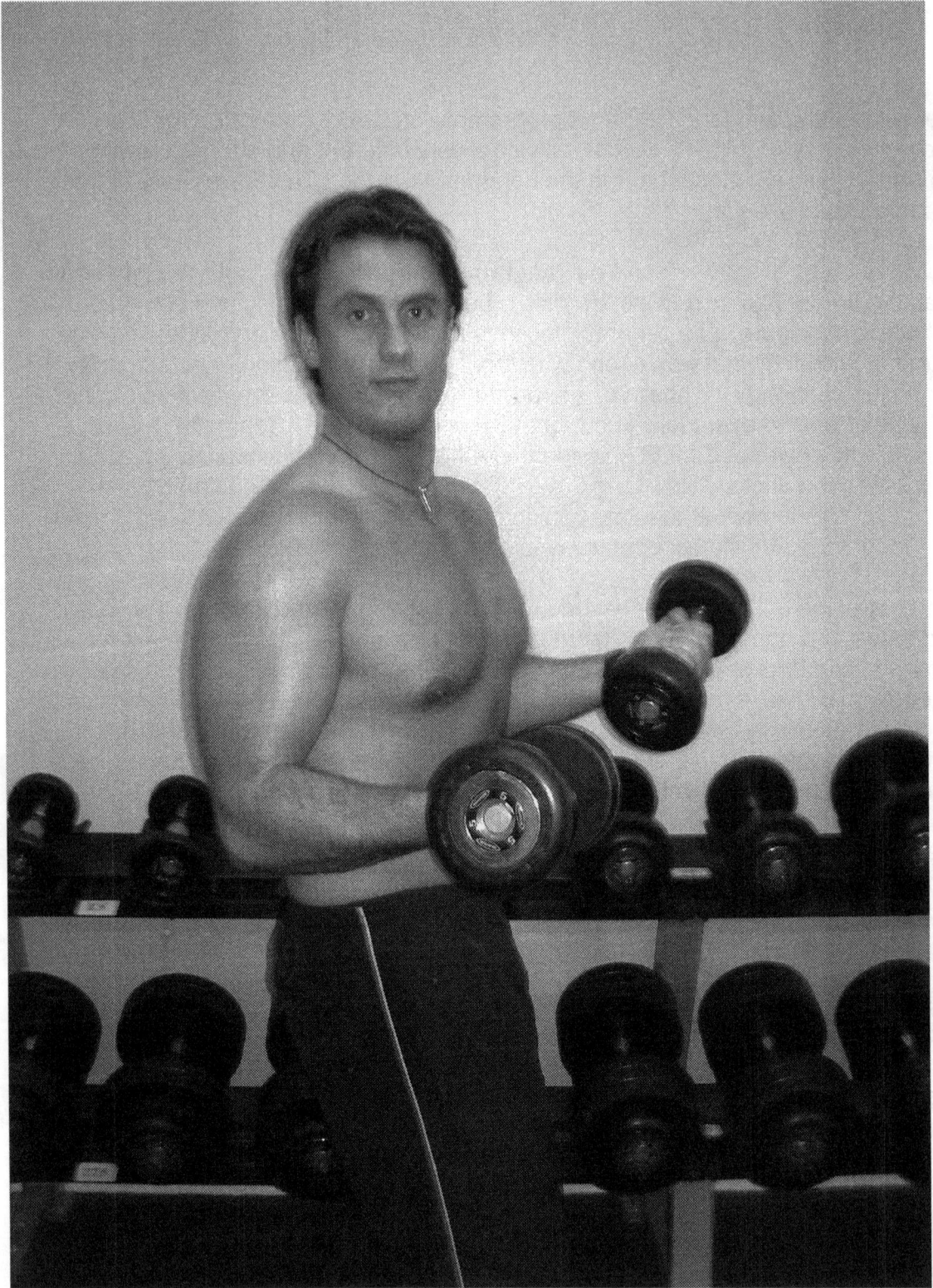

David Tells His Story

I come from a beach resort on the Mediterranean coast of Italy. I have been practicing sport all of my life, especially water-based ones, such as surfing, swimming and canoeing.

Exercise is, without a doubt, my greatest passion and that's why I decided to work within the fitness industry. Exercise gives me the motivation and energy that I need to get on with life and always makes me feel positive. I am convinced that exercise is a lifestyle that can really change people's lives.

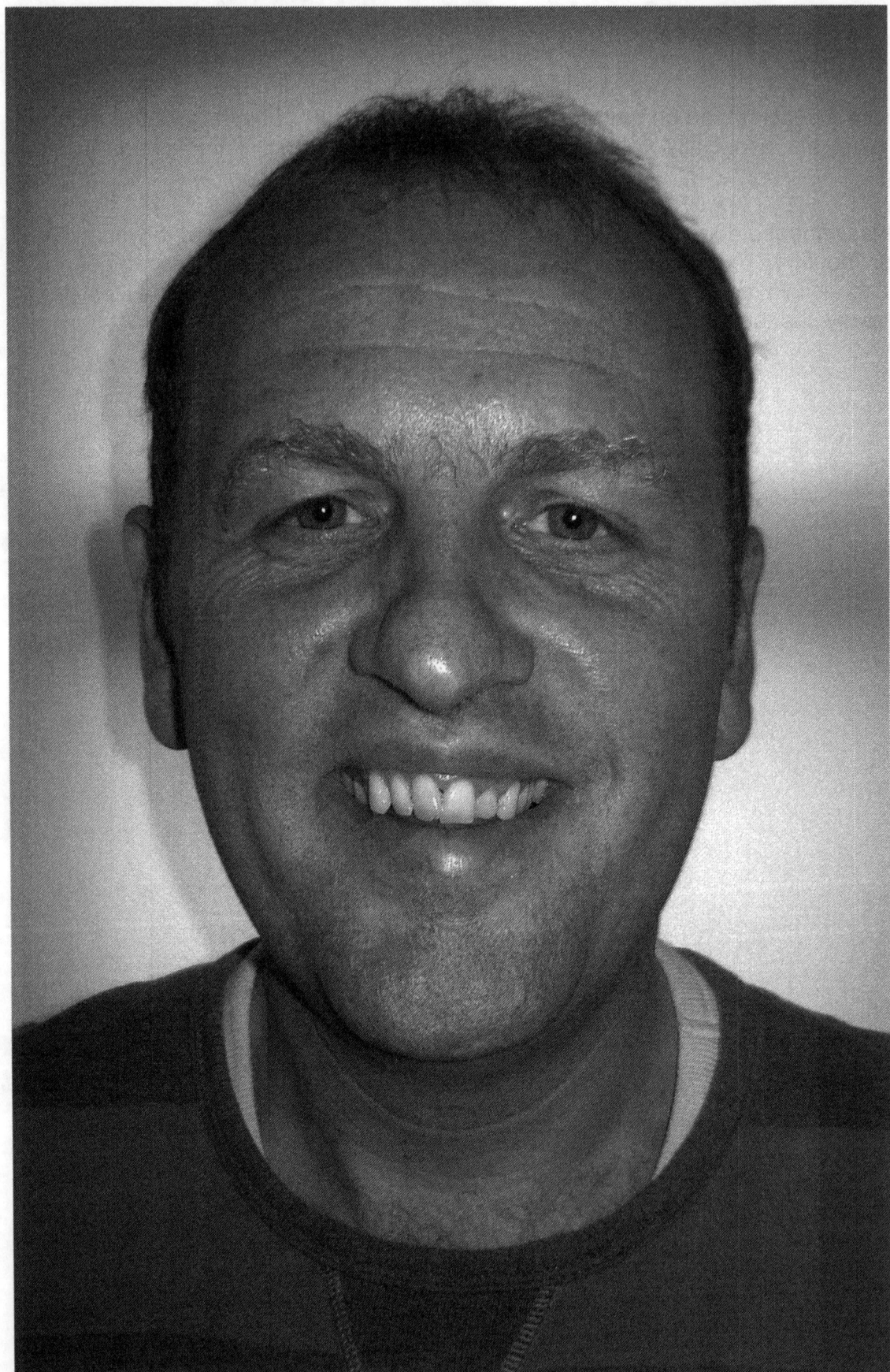

Dean Tells His Story

On the 28th March 2005 our much-loved son, Daniel James O'Hare, aged 19, took his own life. Our family - my wife Shirley and my two sons, Matthew 11 and Ben 7 - are devastated by this tragedy. We moved out of our house and stayed with relatives, as it was too painful to be in our own home, where our son had taken his life. It was obvious that our son Matthew needed professional counselling immediately - he said he needed to talk to somebody - and he was referred for counselling by our GP. It was three months before he received his first appointment. In the meantime, we contacted the Samaritans and a local Samaritan was there for us immediately, at any time, for all the family. It's impossible to describe how I felt at the time that Daniel died. It was as if our lives had been ripped apart. I was prescribed anti-depressants and sleeping pills. The main highlight for me, at the end of the day, was taking the sleeping pill so that I could sink into oblivion and switch off from the pain of our loss.

We wanted something positive to come out of this tragedy so decided, in Daniel's memory, to raise money for the Samaritans. Our two sons designed a wristband to sell, 'IF U CARE SHARE' with Daniel's name on the band. The Samaritans felt this should be a bigger project and adopted the idea with a view to selling wristbands at football grounds. In the meantime I was asked by the local Samaritan lady if I wanted to take part in a BBC programme *Run for Glory* that involved training for six months for the London Marathon and, at the same time, would raise awareness and money for the Samaritans. I thought it was worth giving it a go. I had nothing to lose and it gave me a focus. I was over seventeen stone at the time and not very fit. I'd always enjoyed a game a football but hated running and avoided it as much as possible. I used to look at people out running and couldn't see the point in it. I just thought it was ridiculous.

Before I started training on the programme I was taking beta-blockers, anti-depressants and sleeping tablets. I remember taking my two boys out for a kick around at football and all I wanted to do was lie down, curl up and go to sleep. I had no energy. But I decided to give 100% to the training from day one and within a week I started to enjoy running and feeling good when I pushed myself. I remember the week before I started training for the programme I struggled to run a mile I was so out of breath.

My wife Shirley was, and still is, a wonderful support. She was behind me 100% and made sure that I stuck to my diet. I started to lose weight quickly and lost 4.5 stone in the six months of training. I completed the marathon and it felt so good to reach the finish. I took my last anti-depressant the day before I ran the marathon. This is the fittest I have ever been and I intend to continue running. I have also started cycling to work twice a week (a 20 mile round trip). Nothing will ever stop me feeling the pain of losing my son. I am still grieving, but running and keeping fit has given me so much focus, enjoyment and a sense of achievement. I never went into it thinking it would be a cure but it has given me a big step forward and I am beginning to live my life again. It has also helped the whole family and I have met some wonderful people. I'll never give up regular exercise and hope to continue running. At the moment I am training for the Great North Run and hope to do another marathon. My wife Shirley commented recently, "Now the Marathon is over, can anybody tell me how to remove his batteries?"

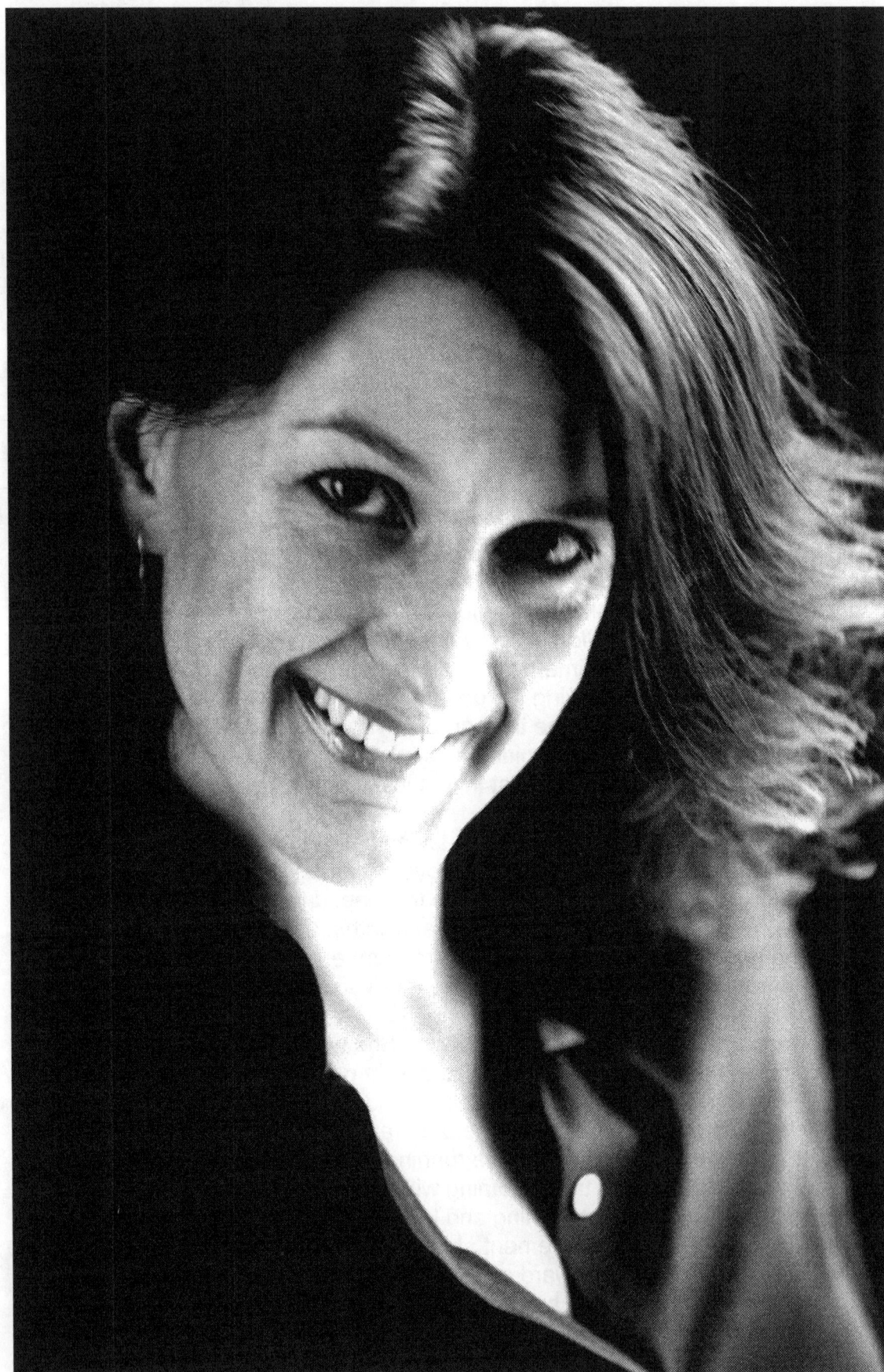

Emma Tells Her Story

I became dissatisfied with my body at a very early age, when I was just eight. I thought that I had a much larger waist than everyone else my age and that my shape was all wrong. My unhappiness lasted throughout my teens into my early twenties, when I eventually reached a state of contentment with my body. By that time I had been practicing Tae Kwon-Do for a couple of years and that had made me fairly muscular and toned. I was still not entirely happy with my body though.

After doing no exercise for a period of about five years, I decided to join the YMCA gym – this was nine years ago - in an attempt to improve my physique and general fitness. It was not until a couple of years ago, however, that I became truly happy with my body after taking up some specific classes that focused on building muscle strength, tone and stamina. These classes included circuit training, weight training and boxercise. It is amazing how, through training specific muscles, you can sculpt your body into the shape that you desire.

I started running two years ago and this has made a massive difference to my overall fitness level. I joined Holme Pierrpont Running Club last year and I am very excited about what the future holds for me in competitive racing. I have a very competitive nature and I love the feeling that you get from seeing yourself improve each time you run and race. I will run my first half marathon this year and I hope to do the New York Marathon next year.

So, finally, after all those years of discontent, I have the body that I have always wanted and, consequently, an increased self-confidence. Another equally important benefit is the great sense of achievement that I feel from seeing tangible results.

I regret very much the fact that I spent so many years being obsessed with food and calorie counting and being unhappy with my physique. I wish that I had discovered sooner the ways in which exercise can transform your body shape. I actively encourage other members of my gym to persevere with their programme, as I am proof that you can achieve your goals through dedication and hard work. I would strongly recommend anyone with a negative self-image to join a gym and discover happiness through exercise. The YMCA gym and Holme Pierrpont Running Club have provided a very friendly and supportive atmosphere for me to train in. For that I am truly thankful.

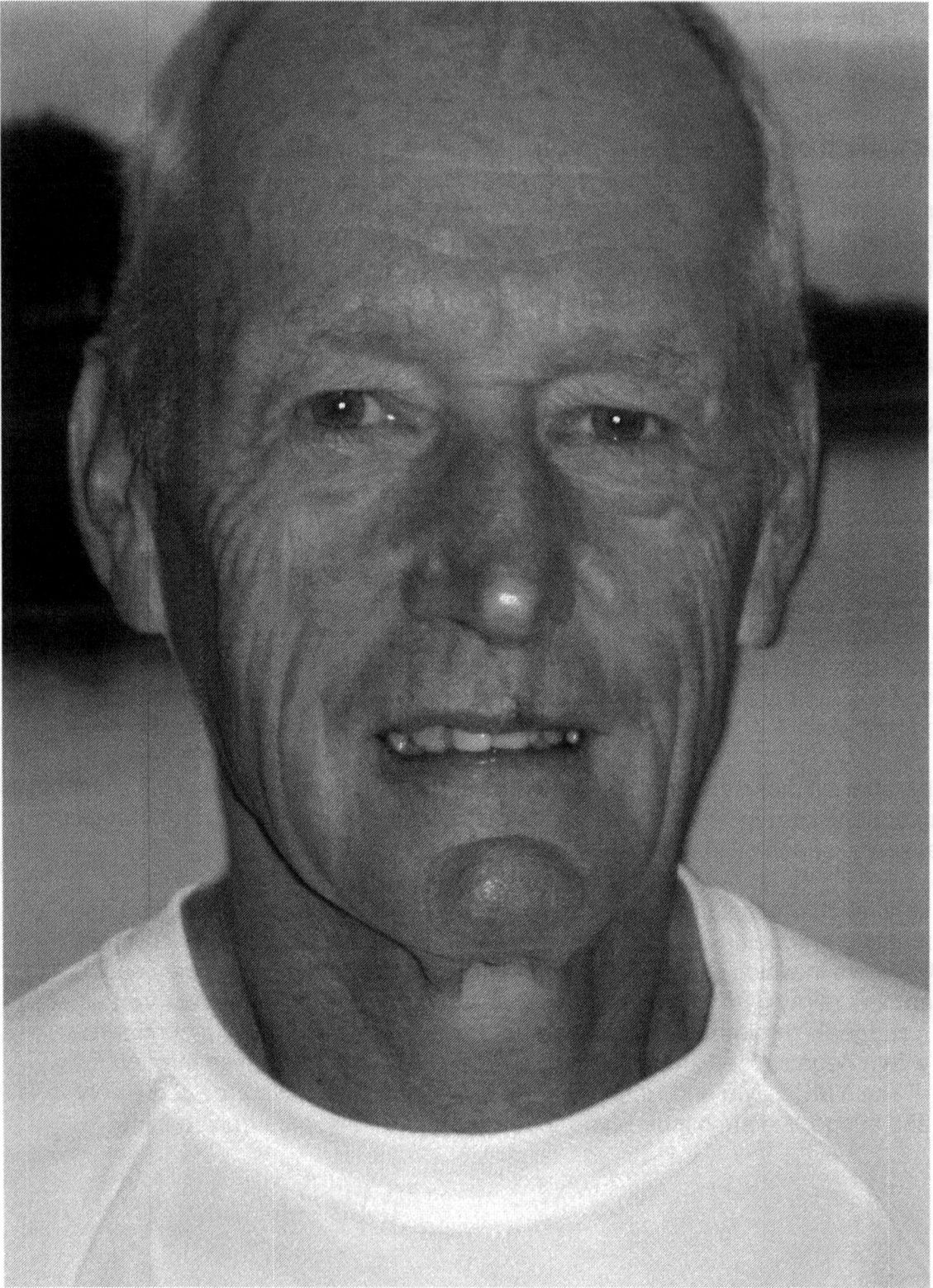

Frank Tells His Story

Since my early twenties I have had a clerical job and was not particularly interested in sport. As my career progressed and my responsibilities increased, I did have some very stressful times, when I became bad tempered at home and experienced difficulty in sleeping.

In 1987 my company sponsored the British team for the 1988 Olympics and I was asked to take part in a twelve mile sponsored run. My training began one night in the dark - so no one would recognize me - and, despite my confidence, I found that I could only run 500 metres before I had to stop for a rest! Over the next few months I gradually improved until I could run five miles in less than one hour and without stopping! Now I was beginning to enjoy running and it was no longer a chore but a pleasure and, more importantly, I found that work worries were soon dispelled once I was out running. I lost weight and felt fit. People also started telling me how well I looked. The race took place on the 8th May 1988. I finished in 1 hour 40 minutes and was delighted. Since that time I have continued running for pleasure. I have joined running clubs and made lots of new friends over the years. My health is good and now in my seventies, I am still running and enjoying the exercise and the good the feeling it brings.

Gemma Tells Her Story

I was smoking sixty a day (more at weekends!) and spending around £50 per night on booze. I was, as you can imagine, very unhealthy. I also took anti-depressants for four years.

I was then diagnosed with cervical cancer and that really shocked me and jolted me into leading a healthier lifestyle. I gave up smoking and started eating healthy food. I joined the YMCA gym and started doing regular exercise. I then got into running, after starting on the treadmill. I recently did a half-marathon in Leeds.

I now feel more confident and, because I feel more confident, I feel more open to making new friends.

Jo Tells Her Story

I have always been a naturally very sporty and competitive person and have been lucky enough to have been able to try many sports, including horse riding, which I now teach. Sport for me is a way of release and escape. I have also found it really useful in making like-minded friends and giving me focus and goals in life.

Just over a year ago I had a total job change, to a more sedentary job and I was really worried that I would start to put on weight as I had previously had an eating disorder in my late teens. This was an issue for me and I found that by exercising I was able to control my eating. Luckily I found the YMCA gym where I formed some excellent friendships and I was able to train and take part in a few more activities, like fencing and boxing. It was then that I realized that I was training very hard but had no goals. I then discovered, by chance, that I seemed to be good on the rowing machine. Seven months later and I am being trained by a former four times world champion, with the hope of doing well in some big competitions.

Being active and sporty makes my life complete and exercise makes me happy!

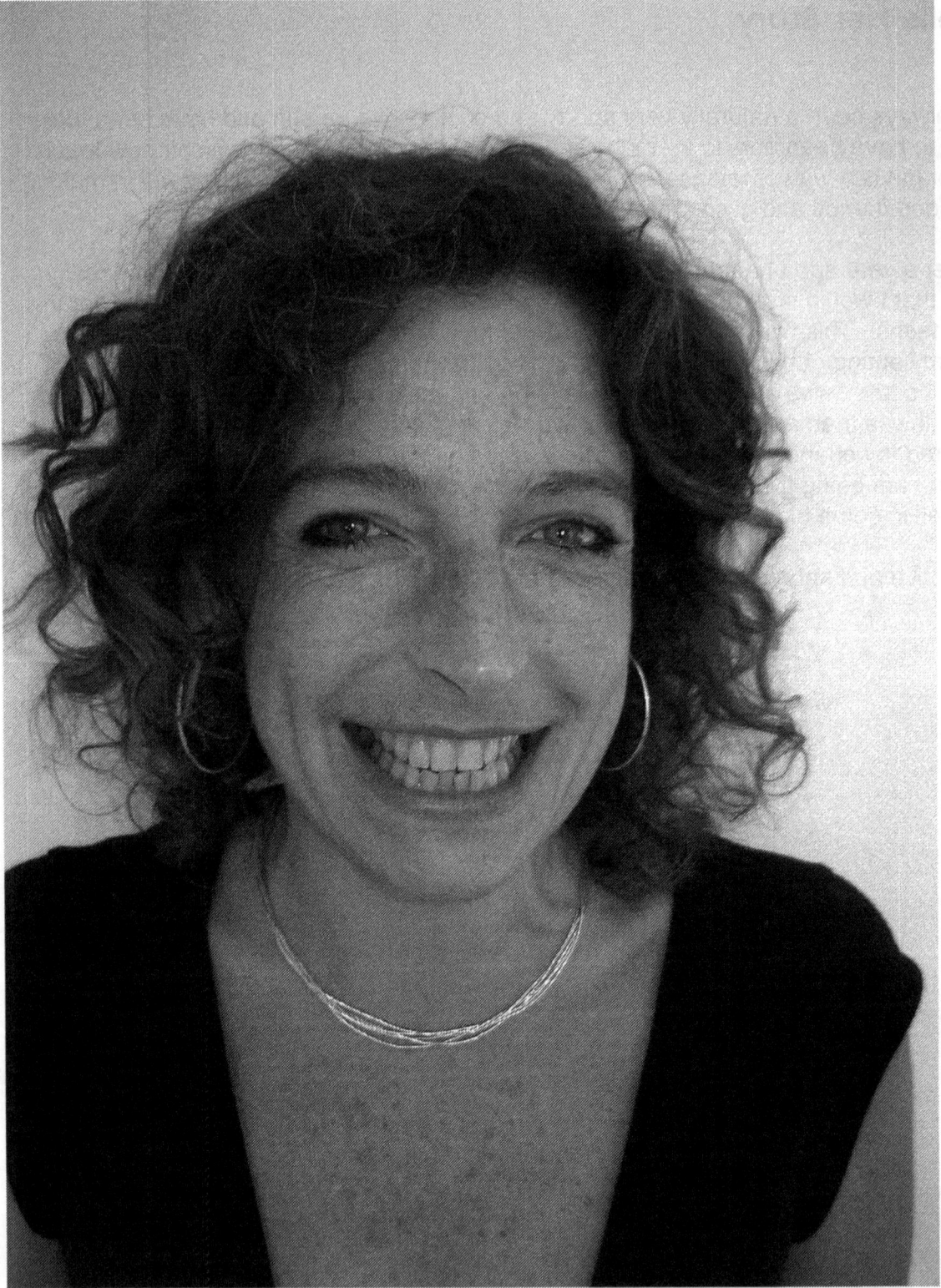

Hilary Tells Her Story

I'd never been good at sports or athletics at school, so I never felt encouraged to try. As a student and a young adult I led a pretty sedentary lifestyle. As I approached forty I had my own version of a mid-life crisis and decided that I needed to improve my fitness or suffer serious consequences later in life. So, I joined a gym, but after six months I was beginning to get a bit bored. It was then that I took up the invitation from another gym member to go for a run. We ran a gentle two miles and it didn't feel too uncomfortable, but it was the praise that she gave me for having achieved the distance that really encouraged me. It made me believe that I could do this running lark and I was excited by the fact that – for the first time in my life – I might be reasonably good at something!

I was quickly hooked and started training for my first half-marathon. I watched the London Marathon on television and was so impressed by the variety of runners – all ages, shapes and sizes – and realized that they were just like me. If they could do it then perhaps so could I. I got a place to run the London Marathon the following year and the added bonus was that it made me feel very positive about becoming forty as I was entering a new age category in race terms.

Running has boosted my confidence enormously. I allow myself to feel proud of completing races and I positively wallow in the awe that marathon running invokes. I also feel the benefits of just going out on a training run. If I have felt low or troubled by something, running has invariably made me feel more positive, or certainly less overwhelmed by it. It has crept up on me, but running has really changed my life. I enjoy the variety of people you meet who are involved in the sport and its accessibility. As it is relatively inexpensive, this means that it is available to all.

Linda Tells Her Story

What made me take up exercise and one of the most taxing of exercises, running? I was pretty unfit, and overweight, and had never done any regular exercise before. I was one of the people chosen to participate in the BBC series *Run for Glory*, to train for the London Marathon in six months.

My young son has Duchene Muscular Dystrophy (DMD) and I thought that by taking part in the programme I would raise awareness of the condition, raise funds into research and also do it in memory of my brother Vaun, who also had DMD and died in 1981, at the age of 18. Neither my brother nor my son would ever be able to run a marathon.

I also hoped that it would increase my self-confidence that has taken a real battering over the last few years. Apart from getting me fit to be able to care for my son as his physical needs grow, I hoped that it would give me an outlet for the frustration, pain, heartache and despair of having to deal with my son's situation.

I found the training really hard, both mentally and physically, but kept going because I couldn't bear the thought of not succeeding. I would have felt such a failure and would have not only let myself down but also my son Daniel, my daughter Helena and my brother Vaun, as well as everyone else affected by DMD. There were times, mainly on the long runs, when I wondered what I was doing and if I was a little mad.

The training has done so much for me. I am a different person to the one I was before. My weight has dropped by over three stone and I no longer dread looking in the mirror at myself. I have more self-confidence and as a result of this, my posture has improved and I now hold my head high. After all, how many people can say they've run a marathon? My fitness is fantastic. I can see such a difference. It used to take me thirty minutes to walk my son to school. Now it only takes fifteen. I now have the confidence that, as Daniel's physical needs increase, I can keep up with them. I also have much more patience with the children, as I don't get as tired so quickly.

Strangely, and I never thought I'd say this, I really enjoy going for a run and I'm looking forward to going on holiday to find somewhere to run! Probably, and most importantly, running has given me the release that I so desperately needed. If I'm having a tough time with everything that's going on and feeling frustrated (it is so hard watching your child slowly die, knowing that there is nothing you can do to stop it) it is great to be able to go out and take it all out on a run. As I run, I repeat over and over what is upsetting me until it's out of my system and back into its place. I come home feeling so much better and, as a result, I am a happier, calmer, more positive person. Being able to run helps me to carry on mentally and to face the future.

Matt Tell His Story

I've always been sporty. I was a competitive swimmer for eleven years. I've done all sorts of exercise: football, rugby, cricket, judo, tennis, badminton and hockey, all at club level.

I used to be really skinny however, and was bullied at school, and up until the age of eighteen I was about 9 stone. I started weight training and through following my own programme, now, at twenty-two, I am 14 stone.

Putting weight on (muscle, not fat!) has made me more confident, both physically and mentally. My whole persona has changed. Building up my body has also built up my confidence.

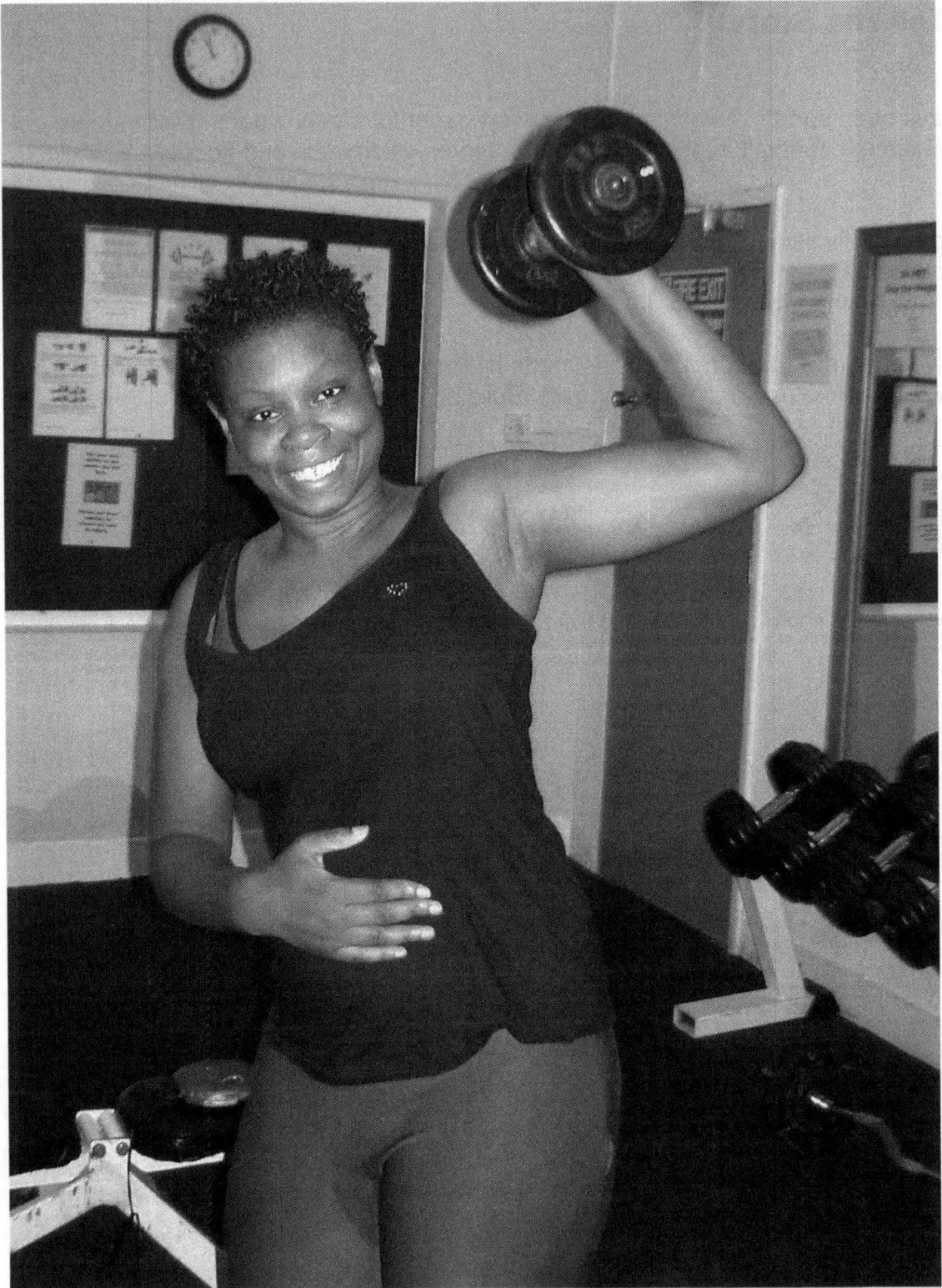

Louise Tells Her Story

About four years ago, in 2001, I had depression and started exercising, hoping that it would help me. I went to a gym twice a week and started to gradually feel a little better after each visit, so I started going three to five times a week and really noticed the benefits. I started to feel so much better. I also lost 3 stone and that did wonders for my confidence.

Not only was I depressed and overweight, I have also always suffered from asthma, which has improved since I started exercising. I used to get around five bad asthma attacks a week. I still have these attacks but nothing as bad as I used to prior to starting exercising. I think my lungs have definitely got stronger from the aerobic exercises that I have been doing. At one stage I couldn't run at all, but now I am able to run for long periods on the treadmill and I feel so much better after a work out.

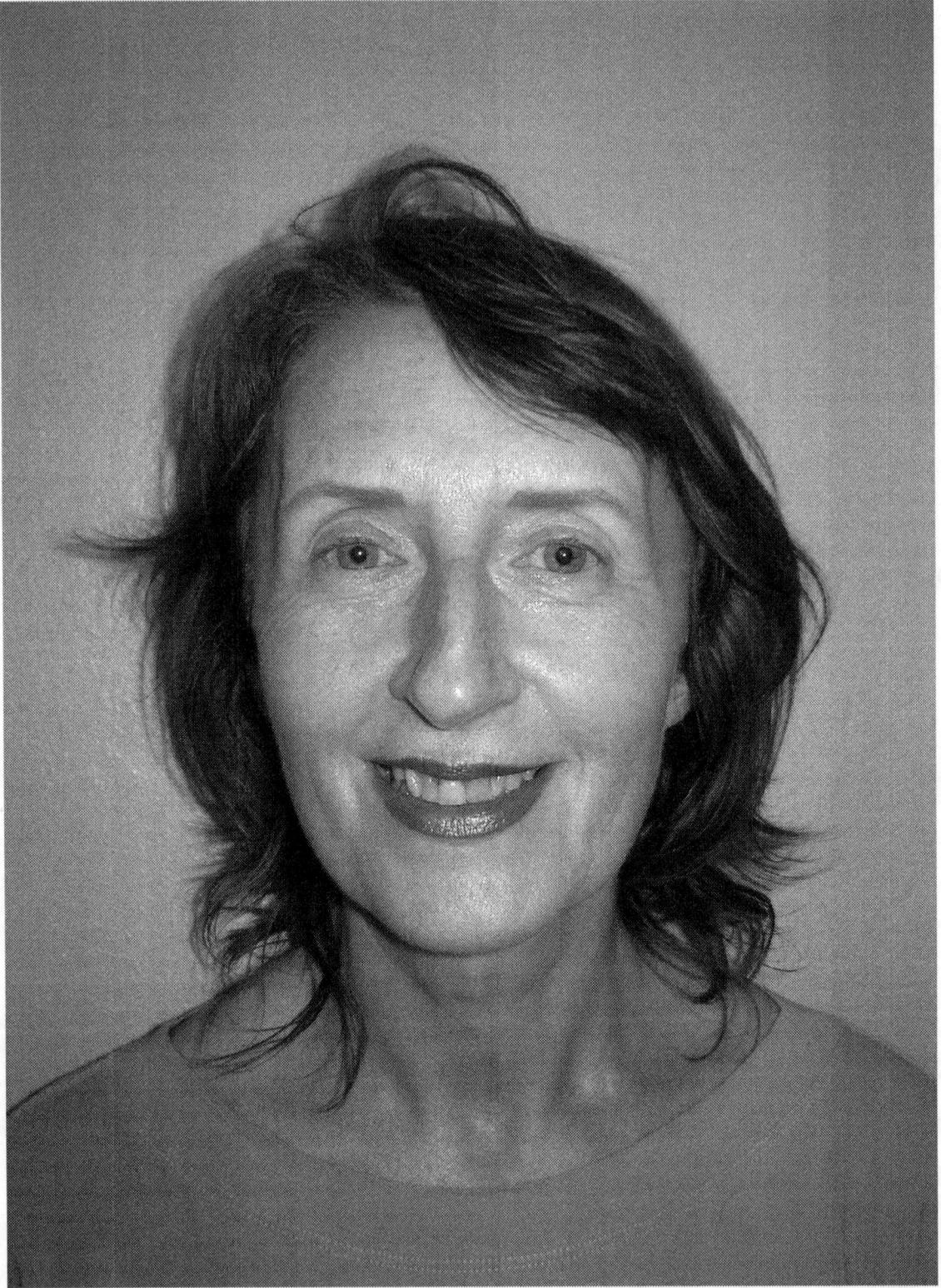

Margaret Tells Her Story

In April 2004 I gave up a very demanding and stressful job as I was beginning to have concerns about my health. In the June of that year my father died and in the July my mother underwent a major operation for cancer and was given months to live. Under the circumstances I became her carer. An episode soon after her operation, when I had to lift her out of the bath, made me decide that I needed to get fitter, not only because of any lifting I might have to do, but to help me cope with the stressful situation.

I became a member of the YMCA gymnasium in the November, not fully realizing how beneficial it would be to me. It's almost a year since I became a member and I feel stronger physically, mentally and emotionally, and friends are telling me that they have never seen me looking so well.

Recently I decided to do some decorating. Painting a ceiling would normally have taken me a few days to complete; with considerable pain in my neck (due to a spinal problem), however the job was completed in hours and without pain.

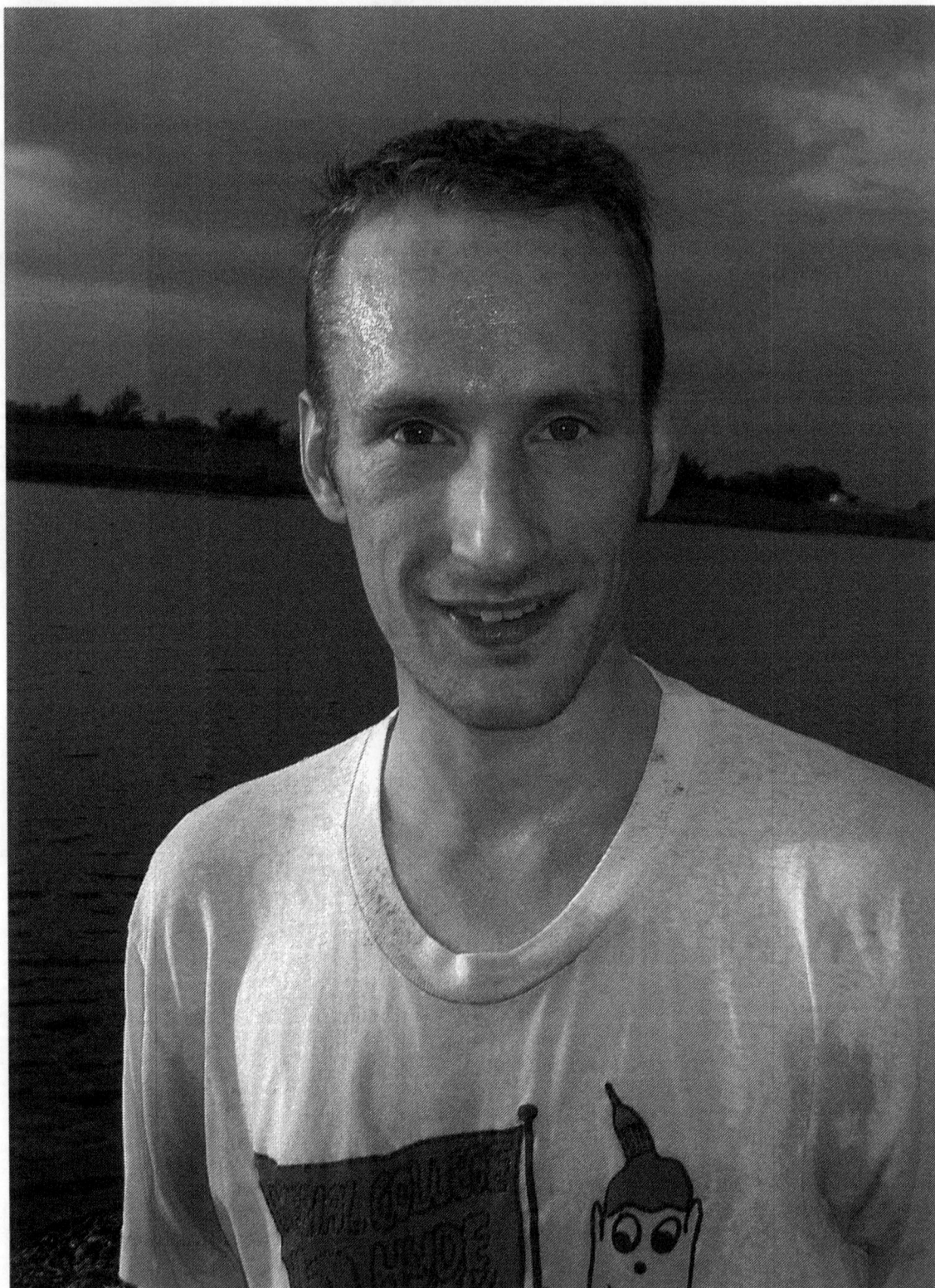

Matthew Tells His Story

I have always been conscious of the physical and emotional benefits of running. Having just completed a PhD, I do not need reminding of what a great stress reliever running can be. For me, however, an additional benefit comes from the increase in self-esteem that comes from finding a sport that I am good at. At school I was never good at football or any other team games and it seemed to take an eternity for me to run 100 metres. Yet when it came to cross country, I always did much better, making school and, later on, county teams. This was important at an age (11-16) when being good at sport was everything.

Being a 'statto' (my profession), I am also excited by the time barriers that us roadrunners face. Breaking one hour for 10 miles and 1 hour 20 minutes for a half marathon were both major achievements for me and, hopefully one day soon, I will add going under 3 hours for the full marathon.

There is no doubt that I will continue to suffer spells of injury and loss of interest, as in the past, however, because of its many benefits and because it is so easy and cheap to undertake, I am sure running will continue to play a major role in my life.

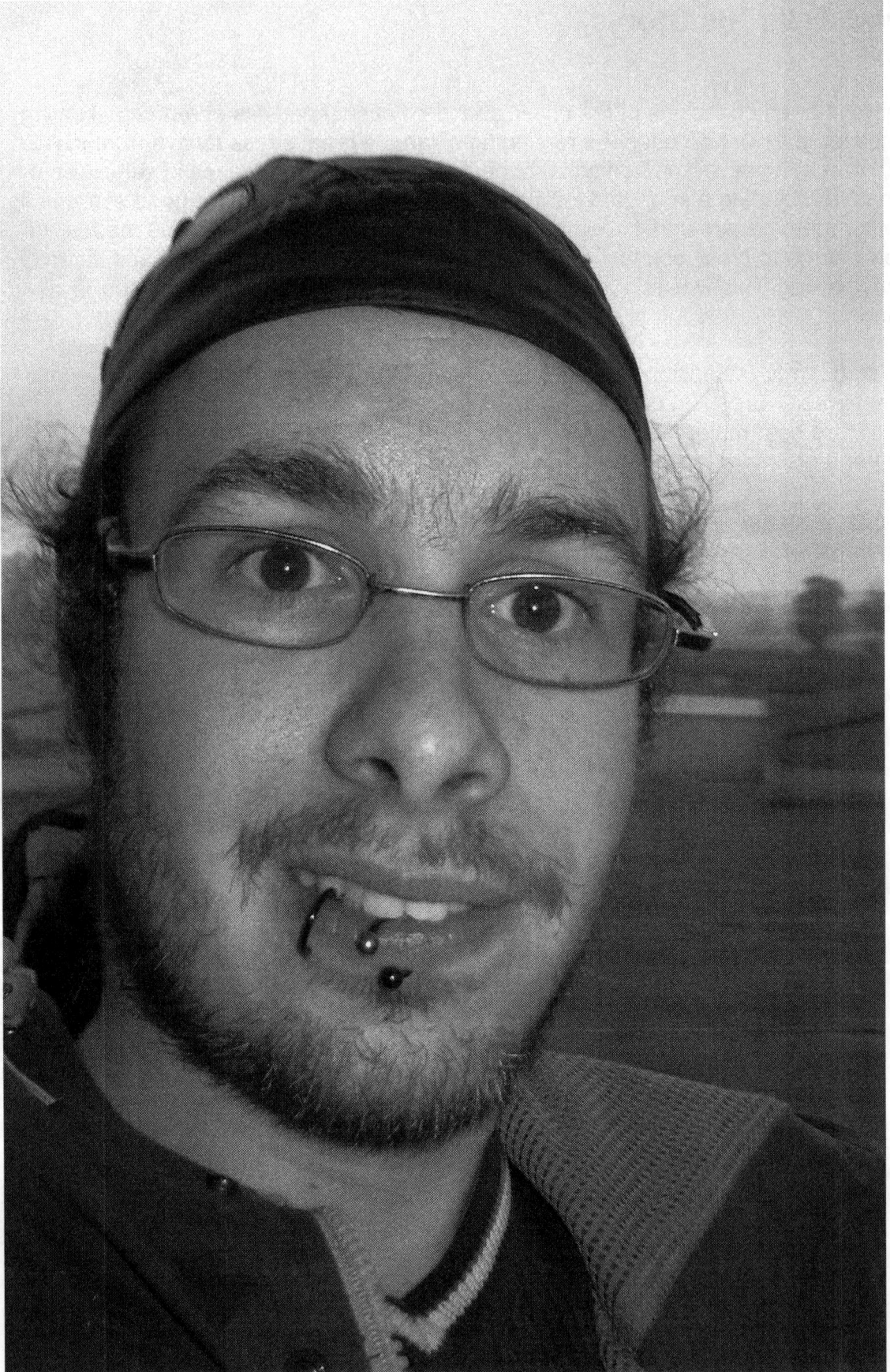

Matthew Tells His Story

Through circumstances in my life I had a serious mental breakdown earlier this year. I even tried to get myself sectioned. I just totally lost control.

Taking up exercise was a great help in getting me back on my feet again. I started climbing and cycling. Cycling is great. I take out my stress and frustrations on my bike pedals! The faster and harder I ride, the better I feel afterwards. It calms me down and clears my head.

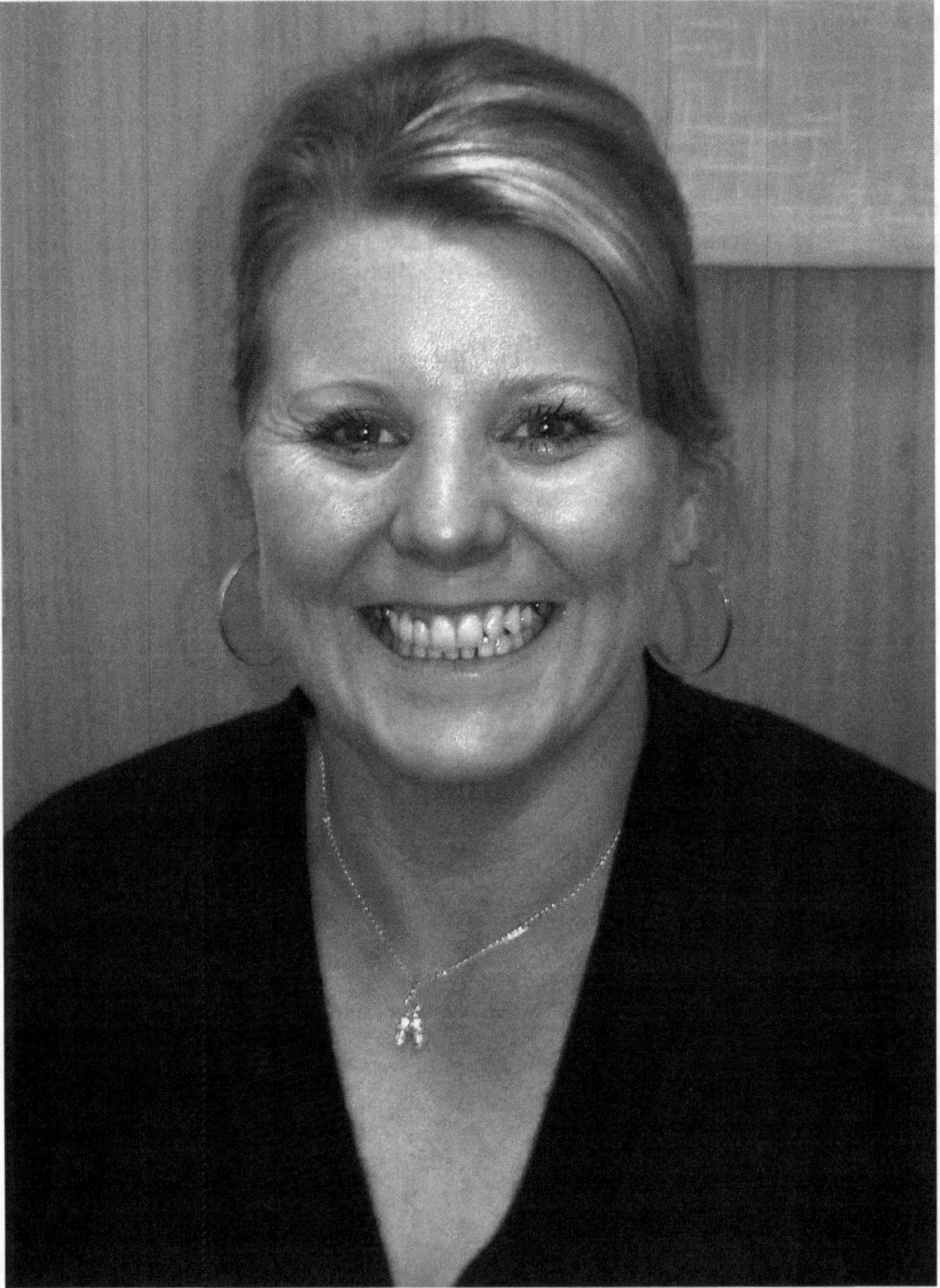

Michelle Tells Her Story

Up to six month's ago I was so very unfit – I was a junk eating, overweight, a smoker (25 a day), and binge drinking at weekends. I had a really sweet tooth and was two stone overweight. The ultimate couch potato!

My dad died at the age of 60 after having a massive stroke at 57, which resulted in his blindness and memory loss. This was a terrible shock. He had smoked 40-60 a day and did no exercise. Instead of learning from this and deciding to give up junk food, smoking and binge drinking I thought *'stuff it'* I'm just going to enjoy my life as life was so short. If that meant sitting in front of the television, smoking and eating junk food, I'd do it. I just didn't think about the consequences.

I didn't grieve properly for my dad and my health began to suffer. I am asthmatic, which was not helped by smoking, and started to get regular chest infections. I also started feeling very depressed. (I have a history of sexual abuse as a very young child). I didn't recognize this as depression as it was the norm for me. I'd been like this all my life. I presumed everybody felt the same. I would often take to my bed and would be literally paralysed with depression. Eventually I went to my GP and I started to take anti-depressants about eight years ago. I still didn't want anybody to know because there is still a stigma attached to depression.

Last year, as a joke, my workmates sent my details to the BBC who were making a programme about a group of people - all with very different stories - training for the London Marathon. I was accepted to participate with twelve other unfit people. We had six months to train. It was so hard but it gave me an incentive. I gave up smoking from day one and also stopped taking Prozac.

I struggled to run at first, even the shortest distance, without getting out of breath, but it got better and I started to enjoy exercise for the first time in my life. I didn't want to give up; I had something to aim for. I lost two stone and felt on such a high after the training sessions.

I did the London Marathon after the six months training and I can honestly say that taking up exercise, and running, has completely changed my life. I feel so much more positive now and want to continue feeling like this. There is no looking back – the couch potato is long gone! I've gone from a size 16 to a size 12 and I feel so much more confident.

I usually do a jog in the morning and feel 'set up' for the day before going to work. I usually do a longer run at the weekend when I'm not working. I now enjoy doing active things with my kids – and they love to see their fit new mum!

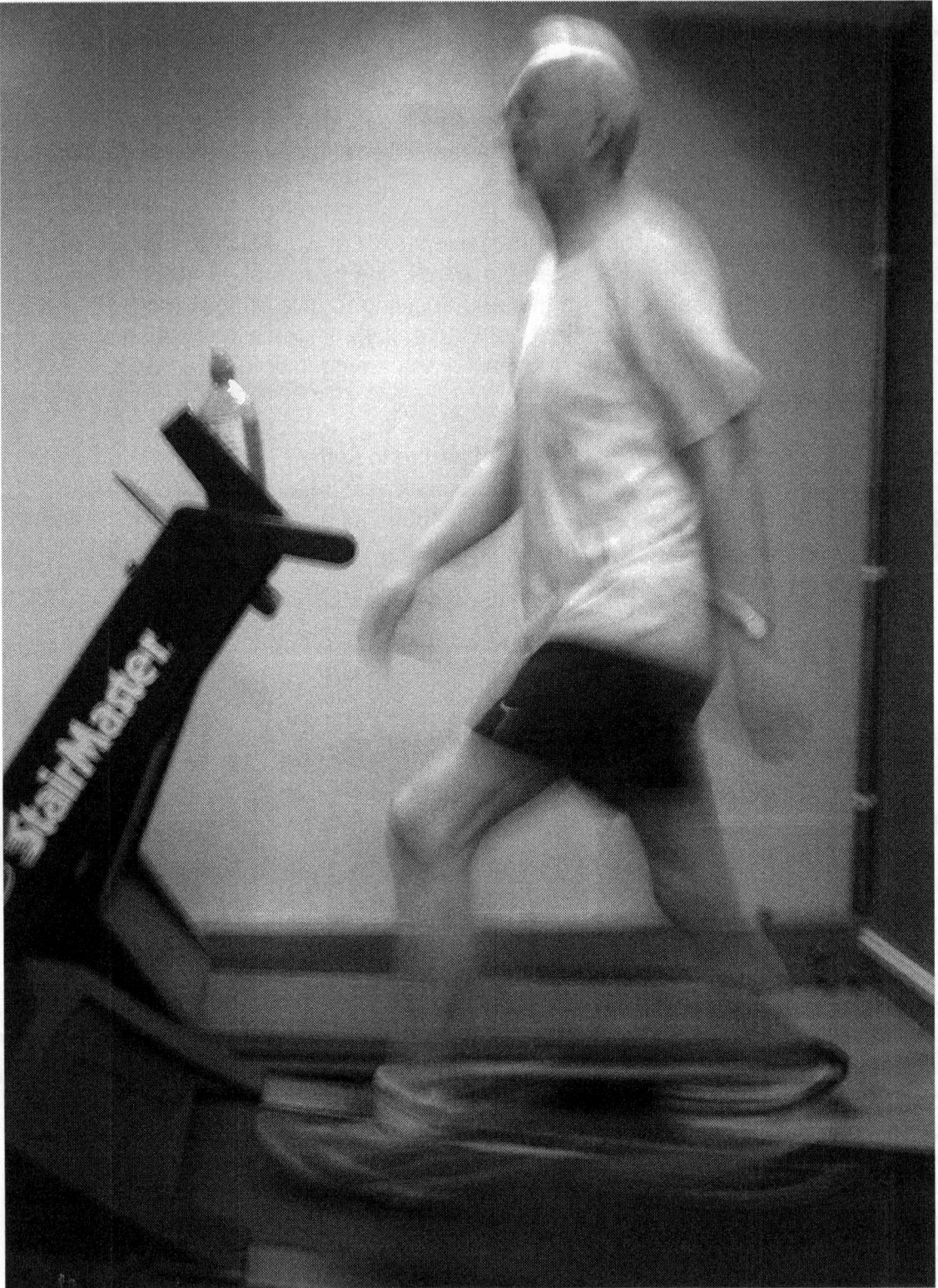

Mike Tells His Story

I've always exercised. I used to run around everywhere when I was a kid. I still run, but I mainly walk now. I am a member of the YMCA gym and enjoy the atmosphere in this gym. Exercise for me has always been a good stress buster. I always feel good after a workout.

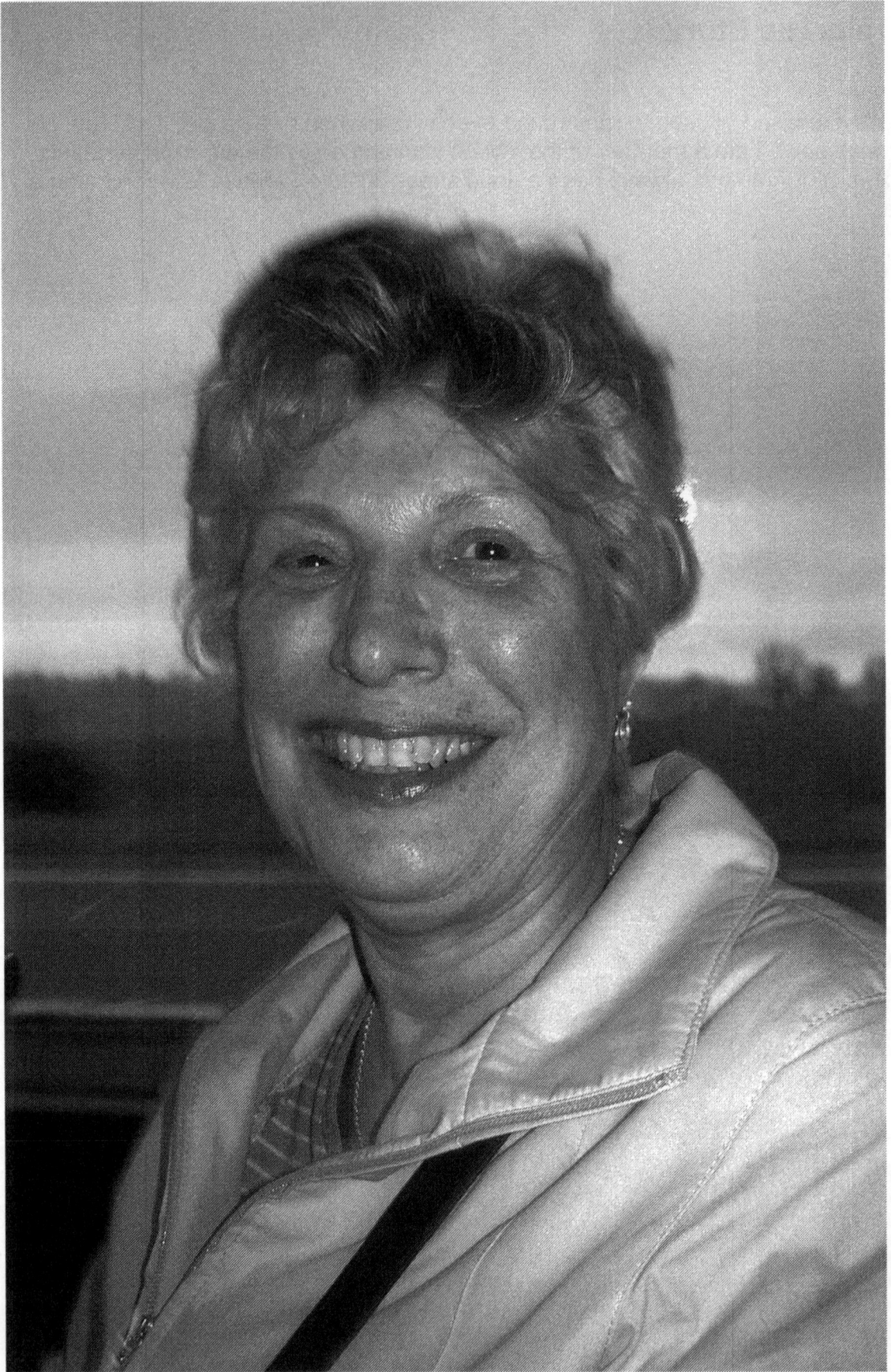

Molly Tells Her Story

I had a stroke six years ago. All of my right side was completely affected. It started to get worse and I was practically housebound. I became very depressed. I had some spiritual healing that helped and I started to get some movement back. I started walking everyday, just a short distance at first. I started to improve physically and I now walk around two to three miles each day.

It feels great being out in the fresh air and I always feel good afterwards. I walk at a good pace and feel uplifted. It makes me feel alive, more alert and my head feels clearer. Walking has definitely helped me mentally as well as physically.

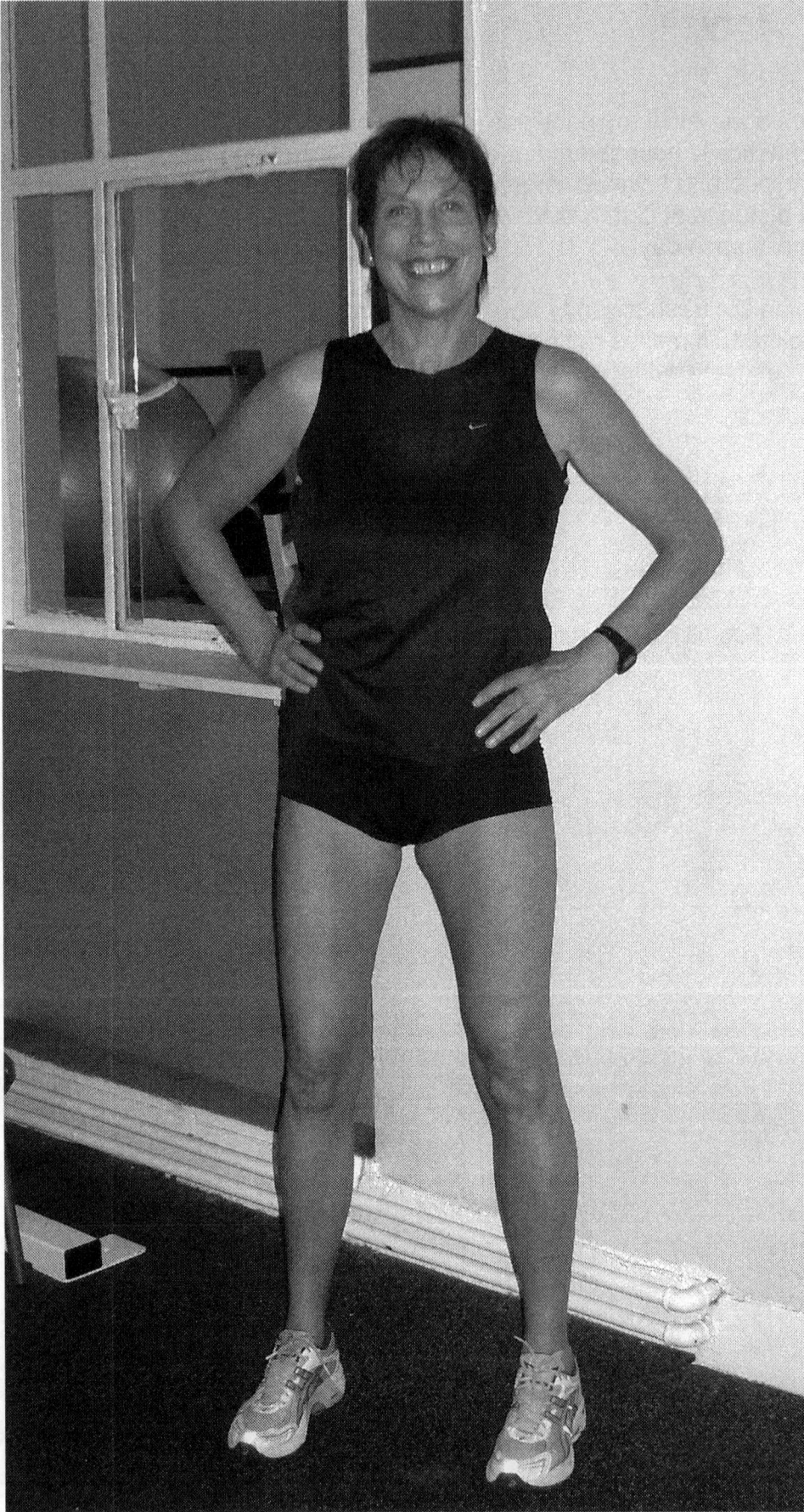

Pat Tells Her Story

Since the age of thirteen I suffered from periods of depression. Due to circumstances in my early life, I had very little self-confidence. It has been a continuous battle, even though I put on a veneer of self-confidence to hide it from others. There have been many times when I would just withdraw into my room and would have to struggle to get through each day. I can genuinely say that regular exercise and training (I took up running quite late in life, just nine years ago) has changed my life.

What made me start? I was going through a particularly bad patch. At my lowest point, rather than resort to taking anti-depressants, hitting the bottle or leaning on others for support, I decided to take up running, as it was cheap. All I needed was a pair of trainers. The hardest part was opening the front door and starting!

I had always managed to keep relatively fit, but never on a regular basis. I had good role models in my parents - they were both keeping active and fit into old age. However, when depressed I would go for months without doing anything. Since taking up running and training at the YMCA on a regular basis, I have chased away the 'black dog' of depression that is always snapping at my heels. Keeping fit has also made me feel good about myself.

I struggled to run one mile when I first started and then started entering races. Racing is the icing on the cake! I have now run thirteen marathons, including London and New York, and I run approximately 20-25 miles a week (30-40 when training for a marathon). I ran my first half marathon in my first six months of running, in a time of just over 2 hours. I have since knocked six minutes off this time. My best marathon time has been 4 hours 9 minutes. Two years ago I entered my first triathlon event and this is a challenge that I hope to develop.

The natural high when you finish a race is fantastic. I can't imagine my life without running now. Training gives structure to my day and I enjoy meeting new physical challenges. My favourite places are to run barefoot on the beach, and through forest paths with the sun filtering through the trees...heaven!

The 'black dog' has never completely disappeared, but when I see it coming, I know I can chase it away!

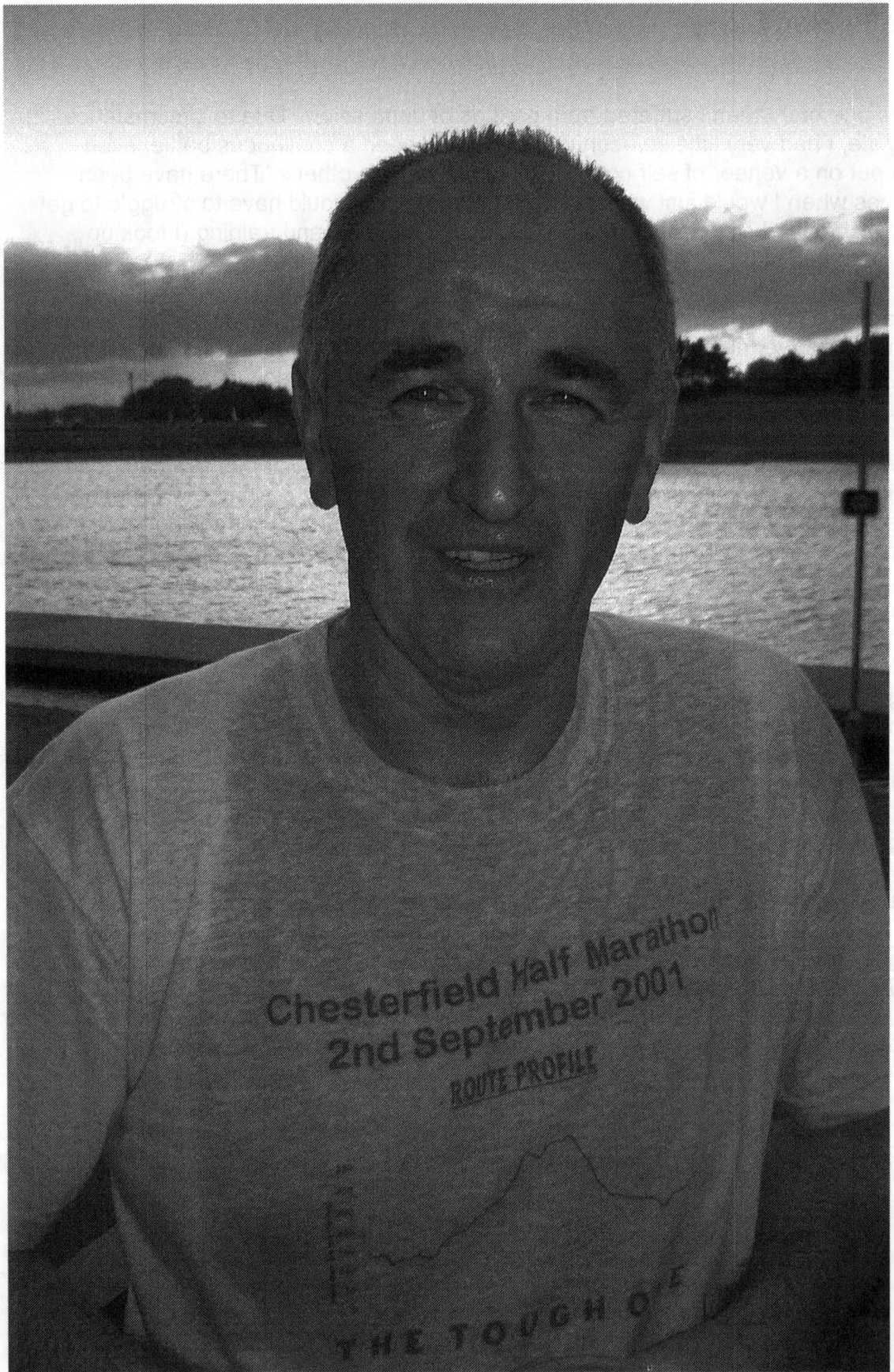

Rob Tells His Story

I was always overweight as a child. Bad diet I suppose. I used to get teased a lot. I was 16 stone when I was 24 and I'm 5' 7"!

I took up running and trained for a half-marathon. I actually enjoyed it, and all you need to get started is a pair of trainers.

I had a very difficult time in my life recently and I handled the pain by training for a marathon. Running has definitely changed my life and increased my self-esteem.

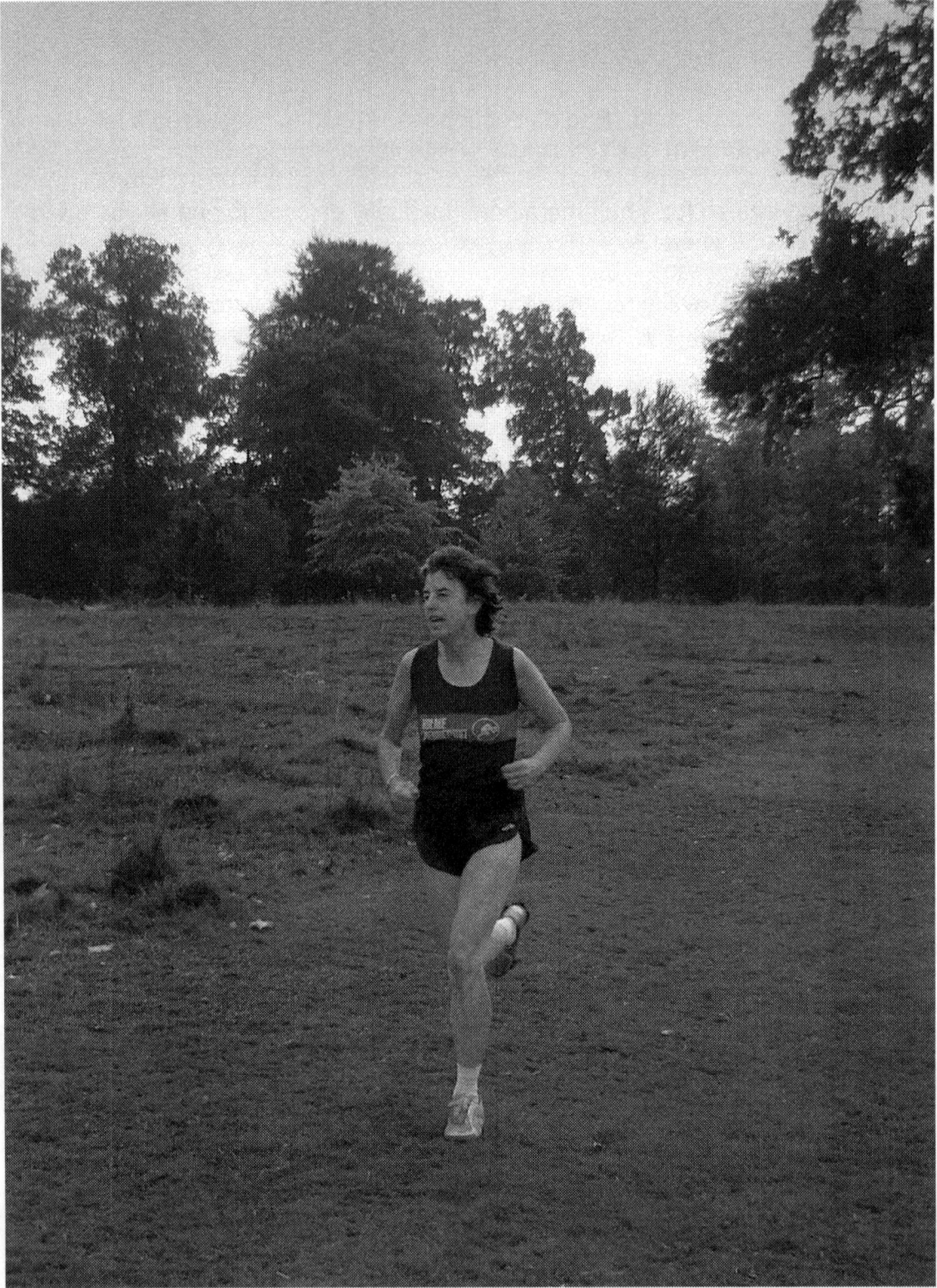

Sandy Tells Her Story

I took up running in my early forties. It wasn't a conscious decision but something that just happened! I went to support my husband on his first marathon and found that by the end of his race I must have run around 9 or 10 miles, on and off, just finding different points from which to shout encouragement. So I started to take it more seriously, first running one mile, then three and onto my first 10k race, which was started by John Denver, the first country singer and, for me, the main attraction of the event.

I kept on running and joined a local running club. Of course I couldn't run a half-marathon, but I did! A full marathon would be impossible, but it wasn't! And that is what running is all about, setting new challenges and meeting them, with all the satisfaction that that brings.

Eighteen years on and now in my sixties, I am still running. Why? Running is one sport where anyone can take part, young and old, and whatever your ability. You can run on your own, or with others; compete or just run for pleasure; run just about anywhere, at any time and in all weathers. The health benefits are well documented and it's a marvellous stress buster and head clearer.

So, has it changed my life? It has certainly enhanced it. Through club events, we have discovered parts of the countryside we'd never seen before and both with the club or just together, we have travelled to many different countries and met a lot of wonderful people. The camaraderie that you find amongst runners is second to none.

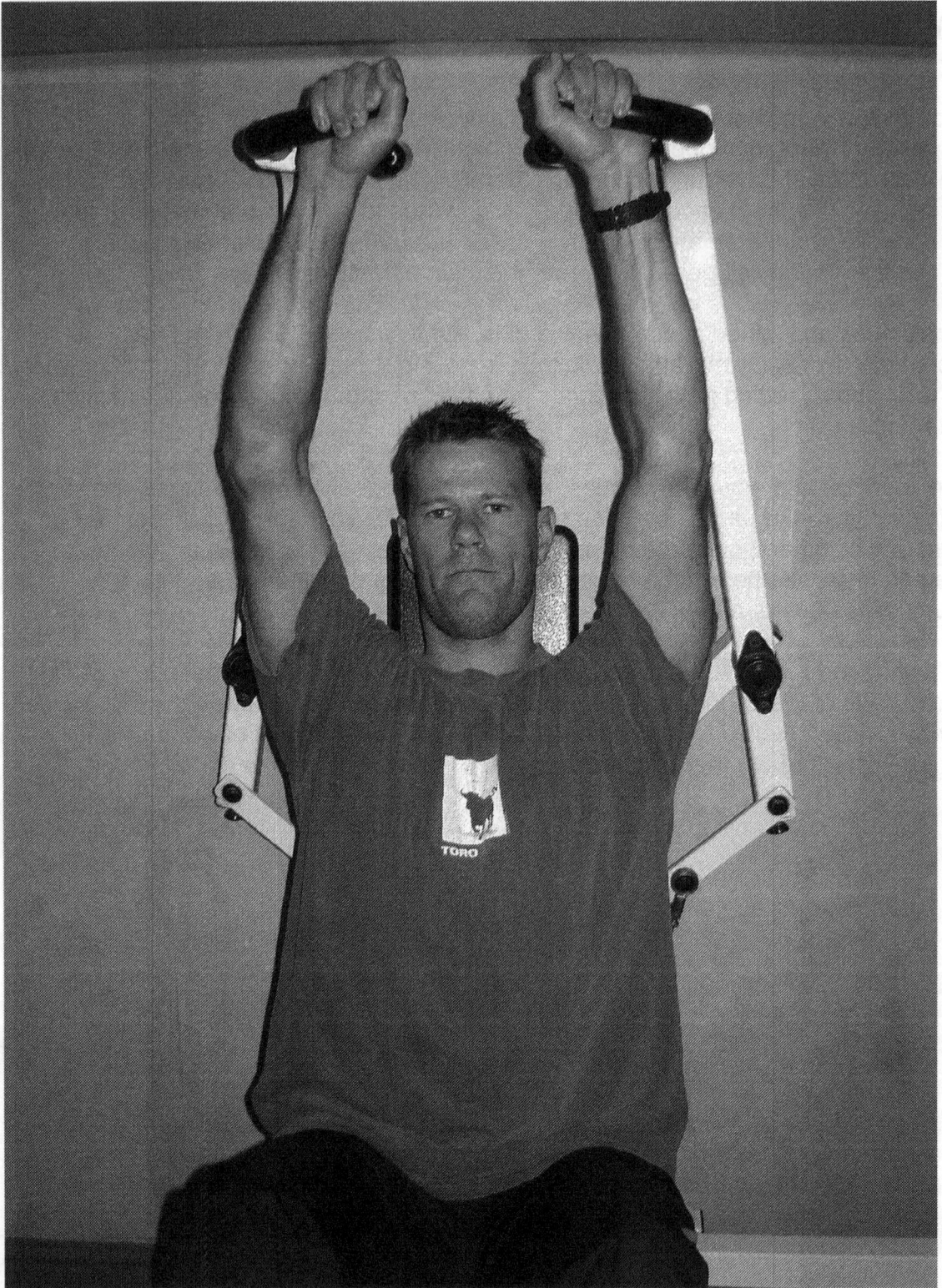

Steve Tells His Story

From a young age I was not a very confident individual. Schoolwork often suffered, as did I within a social environment. As is known, confidence plays a large part in a young person's life and even with encouraging parents, they can't be there all the time. When I was 15 I was invited to partake in a volleyball tryout at school and, as this was a newer sport that hadn't quite developed, I thought, even if I'm not that good, I won't be the only one.

Volleyball was in its development stage within the school and there was a lot of support from coaches and trainers that brought about an excitement that edged you on, to try your best to improve. Others were, as I expected, finding it hard to grasp the skills needed, but nevertheless enjoying the encouragement and challenges put to us.

I think at this point I found the support that I had struggled to find without my family there to push me along. Needless to say, as I kept training I kept improving, my confidence with school and with people followed. I was lucky that I improved so well that I got invitations to play in the national school teams, then local and state competitions.

An improvement in the skills department meant that I was playing with the men, and that meant hitting the gym and getting fit. I had to get stronger, faster and more agile, and had to work hard. My love for volleyball gave me a love for exercise and my love for exercise gave me a love for life. This is something not easily found, but I had never felt more energetic, confident and positive about myself since I joined the gym and started exercising. To this day I still exercise daily, any way I can, and can never look back.

I have had a career in volleyball for thirteen plus years now and have worked in the fitness industry for eleven wonderful years. I have built up my own personal training business in this time and have seen it flourish. I have coached sporting teams to great heights and felt the fulfillment it has bought me. If not for the sport, if not for exercise, who knows what might have become of the young man with little self-confidence? I know of not one of my friends that would have believed for a second that this could have been me.

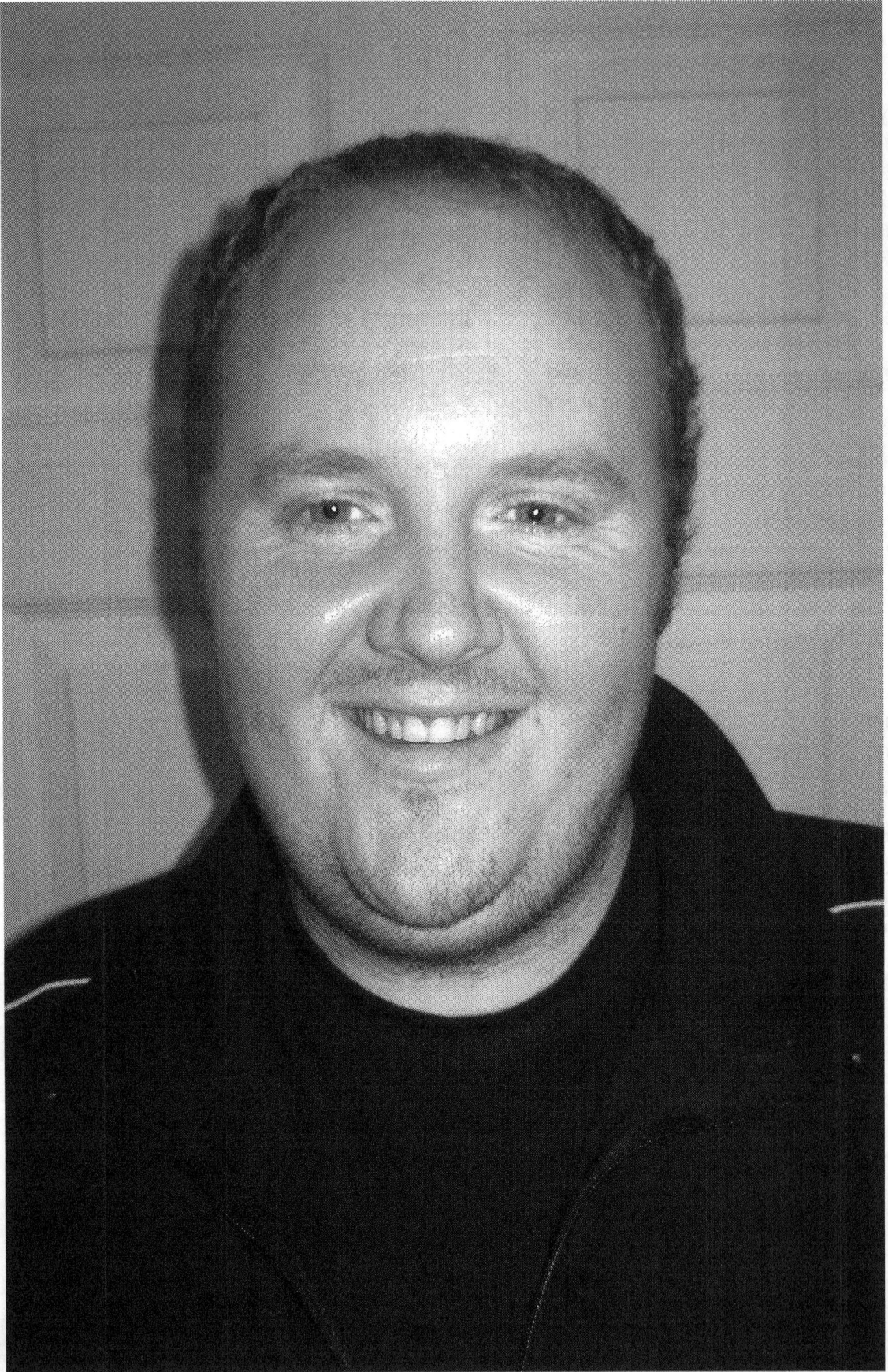

Steve Tells His Story

I was very unfit. I weighed 25 stone 2lbs. I'd been running a football club and always played in goal as I was never able to run around.

Between the ages of 17-19 I'd always be out with a crowd of my mates, drinking most nights and eating junk food. I also like curries, which I had on a regular basis, especially after a drinking session.

I stopped drinking like this when I met my girlfriend Debs. In 2004, Debs, by then my fiancée, died suddenly in the night. Tests were carried out but they could find nothing that had caused the sudden death. I started drinking heavily again after she died. I went to my GP and he suggested that I took anti-depressants and had counselling, but I decided against this. Drink was my way of dealing with the pain of losing my fiancée. I was drinking far more than I did before I met Debs. I reckon I was spending about £300 a week just on booze.

A year later my good friend Andy nominated me for a programme *Run for Glory*, which was advertised on Radio 1. The programme makers were looking for very unfit people to participate in a life changing experience, to train for the London Marathon. I was selected to take part.

It was really hard but gradually, with the weight loss, through exercise, it became easier. I managed to lose 5 stone during training and I hope to continue to get down to my ideal weight of 12 stone. I now eat more healthily and no longer binge drink.

After my fiancée died and I started to put on more weight I thought I'd never meet anybody else who would care for me as much as she did. I had no confidence but running has helped me to believe in myself.

I completed the marathon and it felt so good to finish. I also managed to raise money for my chosen charity, C.R.Y. (Cardiac Risk in the Young). I'll definitely continue running. I've got races booked already this year. I train regularly, mainly in the mornings. I don't run very fast, about twelve minutes per mile, but it feels good to get out in the fresh air and run.

The physical benefits speak for themselves. With this weight loss and the achievement of doing a marathon, my confidence has increased and I think it has opened new doors for me. When I have got down to my ideal weight I am thinking about doing a personal training course for obese people as I can relate to them and say that if I can do it, so can they.

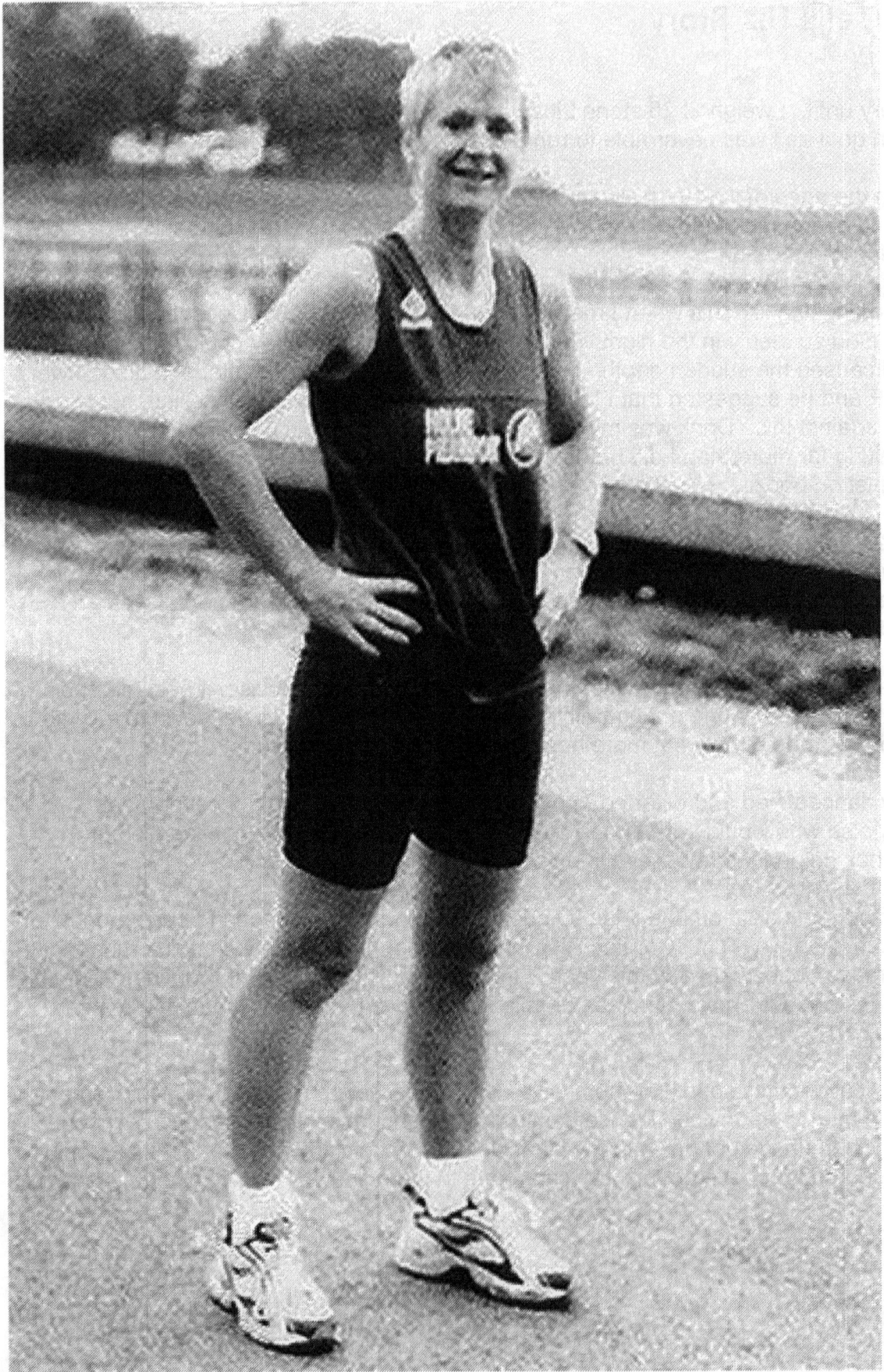

Sue Tells Her Story

I'd always been sporty in my younger days, but after having two children I gained weight and had no time to do any exercise. I lost confidence, my self-esteem was very low and I had fewer friends. Life seemed so boring - just looking after the children, cleaning, ironing, washing and cooking.

After offering to run a playgroup in the village, my confidence started to return and I made new friends, but I still needed to lose the weight I'd put on. So, with three friends, I decided to join a local running club. I made new friends and began to feel better about myself. My weight dropped off me and I felt good.

Exercise, be it running, cycling, aerobics or swimming, is now part of my life. I now have plenty of confidence. Yes, I would say that taking up exercise and making it part of my life has changed my life. Being part of a running club means a lot to me. On my days off I just go for a run and feel loads better. It's an escape from the children! I switch off completely. My friends and family look up to me for the hard work I put in for the various races I have competed in - a half marathon, 10k, fell running, cross country and recently a triathlon event.
This, obviously, makes me feel good and my confidence has increased.

Taking up exercise and feeling more confident has affected other areas of my life too. I've joined various committees in my village and am able to speak out at meetings.

There is a lot of truth in the old saying, "If you feel good about yourself you can tackle anything."

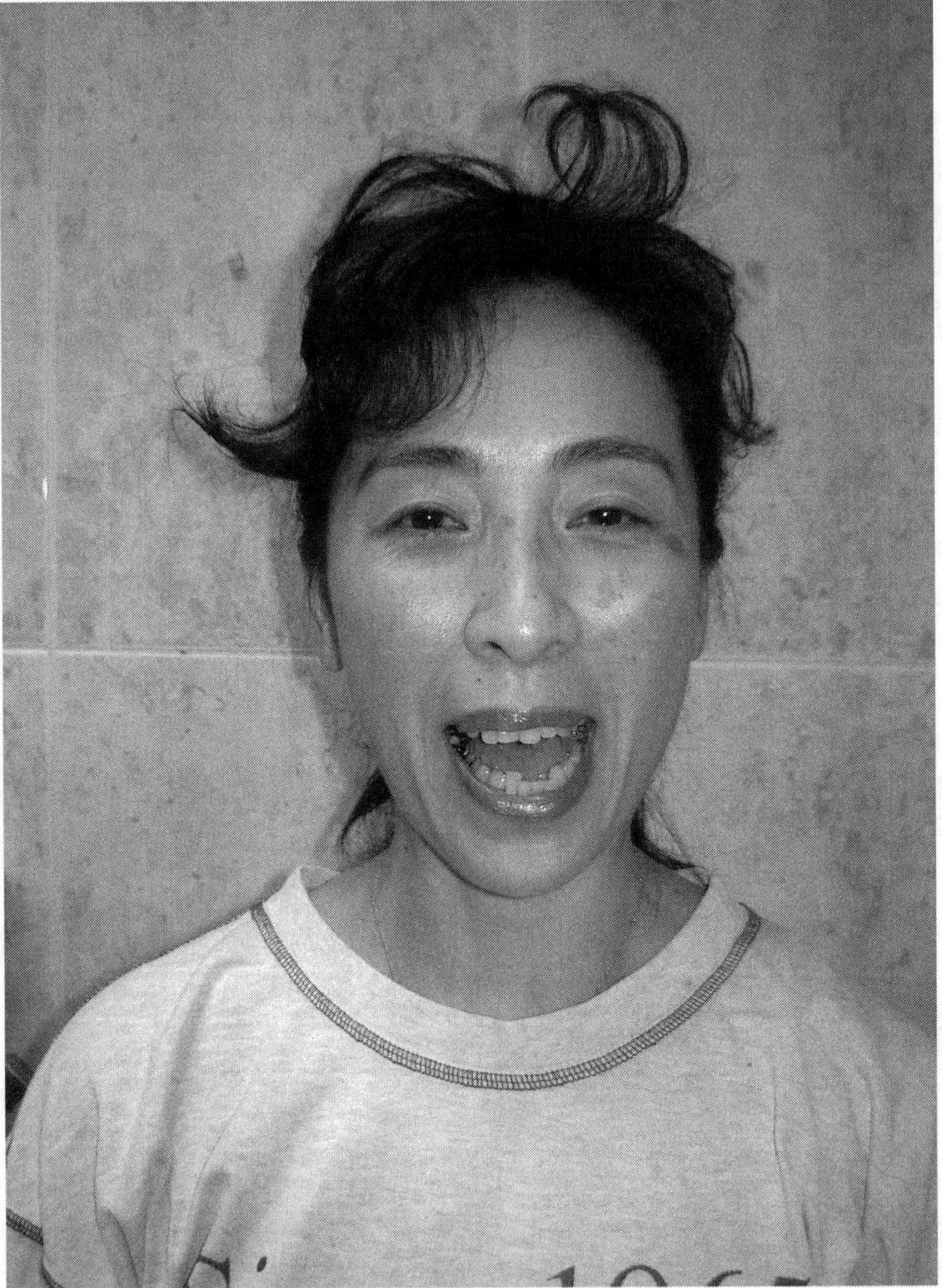

Tomoko Tells Her Story

I came to England from my native Japan to do a PhD. It was very hard at first, not only because of the language barrier (I spoke no English), but I also had to adjust to a very different culture. I knew nobody when I arrived and found it hard making friends because all the other students were a lot younger than me.

I joined the YMCA gym and found that exercising helped me to deal with the stress of adjusting to a completely new environment.

In a gym there are no barriers when you train. Age, culture and language differences are completely irrelevant.   Exercise plays a very important part in my life.

www.ingramcontent.com/pod-product-compliance
Lightning Source LLC
Chambersburg PA
CBHW081508290326
41931CB00041B/3235